Home Care across Europe

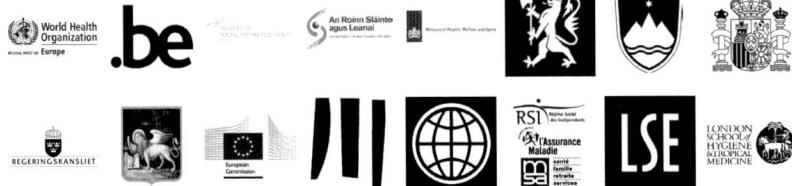

The European Observatory on Health Systems and Policies supports and promotes evidence-based health policy-making through comprehensive and rigorous analysis of health systems in Europe. It brings together a wide range of policy-makers, academics and practitioners to analyse trends in health reform, drawing on experience from across Europe to illuminate policy issues.

The European Observatory on Health Systems and Policies is a partnership between the World Health Organization Regional Office for Europe, the Governments of Belgium, Finland, Ireland, the Netherlands, Norway, Slovenia, Spain, Sweden and the Veneto Region of Italy, the European Commission, the European Investment Bank, the World Bank, UNCAM (French National Union of Health Insurance Funds), the London School of Economics and Political Science, and the London School of Hygiene & Tropical Medicine.

Home Care across Europe

Current structure and future challenges

Edited by

Nadine Genet, Wienke Boerma, Madelon Kroneman,
Allen Hutchinson, Richard B. Saltman

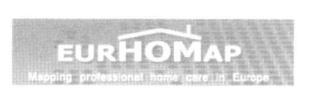
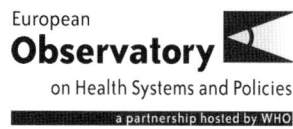

Keywords:
AGED
HEALTH OF THE ELDERLY
HEALTH POLICY
HEALTH SERVICES FOR THE AGED
HOME CARE SERVICES

© World Health Organization 2012 (acting as the host organization for, and secretariat of, the European Observatory on Health Systems and Policies)

All rights reserved. The European Observatory on Health Systems and Policies welcomes requests for permission to reproduce or translate its publications, in part or in full.

> Address requests about publications to: Publications, WHO Regional Office for Europe, Scherfigsvej 8, DK-2100 Copenhagen Ø, Denmark.
>
> Alternatively, complete an online request form for documentation, health information, or for permission to quote or translate, on the Regional Office web site (http://www.euro.who.int/pubrequest).

The designations employed and the presentation of the material in this publication do not imply the expression of any opinion whatsoever on the part of the European Observatory on Health Systems and Policies concerning the legal status of any country, territory, city or area or of its authorities, or concerning the delimitation of its frontiers or boundaries. Dotted lines on maps represent approximate border lines for which there may not yet be full agreement.

The mention of specific companies or of certain manufacturers' products does not imply that they are endorsed or recommended by the European Observatory on Health Systems and Policies in preference to others of a similar nature that are not mentioned. Errors and omissions excepted, the names of proprietary products are distinguished by initial capital letters.

All reasonable precautions have been taken by the European Observatory on Health Systems and Policies to verify the information contained in this publication. However, the published material is being distributed without warranty of any kind, either express or implied. The responsibility for the interpretation and use of the material lies with the reader. In no event shall the European Observatory on Health Systems and Policies be liable for damages arising from its use. The views expressed by authors, editors, or expert groups do not necessarily represent the decisions or the stated policy of the European Observatory on Health Systems and Policies or any of its partners.

ISBN 978 92890 02882

Printed in the United Kingdom

Cover design by M2M

Contents

Preface	vii
List of tables, figures and boxes	xi
List of abbreviations	xiii

Chapter 1 Introduction and background — 1
Wienke Boerma, Nadine Genet

1.1	Objective and structure of this book	1
1.2	Challenges of home care in Europe	2
1.3	Definition of home care	9
1.4	Conceptual framework	10
1.5	Problem and research questions	13
1.6	Methods	13
1.7	What was known about home care in Europe	15
1.8	What this book adds to the current knowledge	20

Chapter 2 The policy perspective — 25
Nadine Genet, Madelon Kroneman, Carlos Chiatti, László Gulácsi, Wienke Boerma

2.1	Policy challenges in the European home-care sector	25
2.2	Governance by European governments	27
2.3	Governance on home-care funding	39
2.4	Challenges and developments	50

Chapter 3 Clients in focus — 55
Vjenka Garms-Homolovà, Michel Naiditch, Cecilia Fagerström, Giovanni Lamura, Maria Gabriella Melchiorre, László Gulácsi, Allen Hutchinson

3.1	Introduction	55
3.2	Clients	56
3.3	Access to home care	58
3.4	Informal caregivers and their role in the care process	63
3.5	Challenges and developments	66

Chapter 4 Management of the care process   **71**
Nadine Genet, Allen Hutchinson, Michel Naiditch, Vjenka Garms-Homolová, Cecilia Fagerström, Maria Gabriella Melchiorre, Madelon Kroneman, Cosetta Greco

4.1	Introduction	71
4.2	Who provides home care?	71
4.3	Integrated home-care delivery	76
4.4	Human resources	84
4.5	Telecare	90
4.6	Quality monitoring, management and improvement	90
4.7	Challenges and developments	97
4.8	Overview and policy issues	102

Chapter 5 Conclusions and the way forward   **105**
Nadine Genet, Wienke Boerma, Madelon Kroneman, Allen Hutchinson

5.1	Complexity of the home-care sector	105
5.2	Taking on the challenge	108
5.3	System-tailored responses to challenges	113
5.4	Ways forward: the EU perspective	120
5.5	Options for policy-makers	120
5.6	In conclusion	122

Appendix I	**Terminology**	**123**
Appendix II	**Case narratives (vignettes)**	**125**

Preface

This book, consisting of two volumes, is the result of the EURHOMAP (Mapping Professional Home Care in Europe) study that was carried out from 2008 until 2010. The project was developed and coordinated by the Netherlands Institute for Health Services Research in collaboration with other researchers and their institutes in European countries. All members of this partnership have contributed to this book by gathering data and writing a chapter or reviewing the book. Their names and affiliations are listed below.

Netherlands Institute for Health Services Research (NIVEL), Utrecht, the Netherlands: Wienke Boerma, Nadine Genet, Dionne Sofia Kringos and Madelon Kroneman

University of Sheffield, Sheffield, United Kingdom: Allen Hutchinson

Blekinge Institute of Technology, School of Health Sciences, Karlskrona, Sweden: Ania Willman and Cecilia Fagerström

Jordi Gol Institute for Research in Primary Care (IDIAP), Barcelona, Spain: Bonaventura Bolibar

National Institute of Health and Science on Ageing (INRCA), Ancona, Italy: Giovanni Lamura, Maria Gabriella Melchiorre, Cosetta Greco and Carlos Chiatti

Corvinus University, Budapest, Hungary: László Gulácsi

Institute for Research and Information in Health Economics (IRDES), Paris, France: Michel Naiditch

Medical University of Bialystok, Bialystok, Poland: Sławomir Chlabicz

Alice Salomon University of Applied Sciences, Berlin, Germany: Vjenka Garms-Homolovà

The partnership is greatly indebted to the experts in each country who have contributed to the data and information on which this study is based. The names and affiliations of the country experts that agreed to be mentioned are listed with the country reports that can be found in Volume II (online only) of this book and on the web site (www.nivel.eu/eurhomap).

Austria. *Vjenka Garms-Homolovà*
Belgium. *Michel Naiditch, Nadine Genet, Wienke Boerma*
Bulgaria. *Nadine Genet, Wienke Boerma*
Croatia. *László Gulácsi, Vanessa Benkovic*
Cyprus. *Nadine Genet, Wienke Boerma*
Czech Republic. *Vjenka Garms-Homolová*
Denmark. *Cecilia Fagerström, Ania Willman*
England. *Allen Hutchinson*
Estonia. *Kaja Polluste, Sławomir Chlabicz*
Finland. *Nadine Genet, Wienke Boerma, Sari Rissanen*
France. *Michel Naiditch*
Germany. *Vjenka Garms-Homolová*
Greece. *Elizabeth Mestheneos, Giovanni Lamura*
Hungary. *László Gulácsi, Adrienn Ujváriné Siket, Gabriella Csillik, József Betlehem*
Iceland. *Allen Hutchinson*
Ireland. *Allen Hutchinson*
Italy. *Maria Gabriella Melchiorre, Cosetta Greco, Maria Lucchetti, Carlos Chiatti, Giovanni Lamura*
Latvia. *Nadine Genet, Wienke Boerma*
Lithuania. *Arvydas Seskevicius, Jurgita Grigiene, Sławomir Chlabicz*
Luxembourg. *Nadine Genet, Wienke Boerma*
Malta. *Joseph Troisi, Giovanni Lamura*
Netherlands. *Nadine Genet, Wienke Boerma*
Norway. *Cecilia Fagerström, Ania Willman*
Poland. *Sławomir Chlabicz, Ludmila Marcinowicz, Wieslawa Mojsa*
Portugal. *Silvina Santana, Patrícia Redondo, Nina Szczygiel*
Romania. *László Gulácsi, Livia Popescu*
Slovakia. *Nadine Genet, Wienke Boerma*
Slovenia. *Nadine Genet, Simona Smolej, Wienke Boerma*
Spain. *Bonaventura Bolibar, Angels Ondiviela, Joan Carles Contel-Segura, Carme Lacasa, Anna Moleras, Joana Maria Taltavull, José Miguel Morales, Isabel Blasco*
Sweden. *Cecilia Fagerström, Ania Willman*
Switzerland. *Michel Naiditch, Elisabeth Hirsch Duret*

The study has been funded by the European Commission (DG SANCO).

Finally, we extend our gratitude to the external reviewers of the manuscript of this book: Chris Paley (HomeCare Europe; National Homecare Council, England) and Professor Jouke van der Zee (Faculty of Health Sciences, University of Maastricht, the Netherlands). Their critical reading and their suggestions have considerably improved our text. Finally we would like to thank Jonathan North and Caroline White, as well as Peter Powell (typesetting), Jo Woodhead (editing) and Sarah Cook (proofreading).

Appendix I defines the terminology used in the book. Appendix II provides the case narratives (vignettes) that have been used as instruments in this study.

The editors

suggestions have considerably improved our text. Finally we would like to thank Jonathan North and Caroline White, as well as Peter Powell (typesetting), Jo Woodhead (editing) and Sarah Cook (proofreading).

Appendix I defines the terminology used in the book. Appendix II provides the case narratives (vignettes) that have been used as instruments in this study.

The editors

List of tables, figures and boxes

Tables

Table 2.1	Fragmentation of home-care policy	30
Table 2.2	Strength of national governmental control over the home-care sector	32
Table 2.3	Overall level of (national) governance for setting a vision, involvement in regulation and integration of home-care policy	36
Table 2.4	Three main types of home-care governance	38
Table 2.5	Number of home-care services receiving public funding	42
Table 2.6	Funding of formal home care	46
Table 4.1	Ownership of home-care providers and the existence of competition in 31 European countries	74
Table 4.2	Models of integration for home health and social home care	77
Table 4.3	Integration of home-care delivery throughout Europe	78
Table 4.4	Integration of home-care delivery with other types of care	81
Table 4.5	Indications for the quality of human resources	87
Table 4.6	Three broad models of quality management	98
Table 5.1	Challenges in home care: responses and their possible consequences	114
Table 5.2	Typology of home-care systems: different challenges and solutions	117

Figures

Fig. 1.1	Preference for professional home-care and opinion on affordability of home care	4
Fig. 1.2	Old-age dependency ratio in Europe, 2010 and 2050	7
Fig. 1.3	Self-perceived limitations in daily activities of retired people in Europe	8
Fig. 1.4	Conceptual framework	12
Fig. 2.1	Home-care expenditures as a proportion of GDP	45

Boxes

Box 4.1	Innovative ways of dealing with human resource shortages	89

List of abbreviations

ADI	Servizio di Assistenza Domiciliare Integrata (integrated home-care service)
ADL	activities of daily living
ANESM	Agence nationale de l'évaluation et de la qualité des établissements et des services sociaux et médico-sociaux
CQC	Care Quality Commission
EU	European Union
GDP	gross domestic product
GP	general practitioner
IADL	instrumental activities of daily living
IGZ	Health Care Inspectorate (Netherlands)
NGO	nongovernmental organization
NIVEL	Netherlands Institute for Health Services Research
OECD	Organisation for Economic Co-operation and Development

Chapter 1
Introduction and background

Wienke Boerma, Nadine Genet

1.1 Objective and structure of this book

The scarcity of up-to-date and comparative information on home care in Europe is in contrast to the growing size and importance of the sector. This book aims to respond to a need for this information as reflected inter alia in the 2006 Public Health Work Plan of the European Commission.[1] No further overview has been published since a study on the organization and financing of home care in 15 countries published in 1996 (Hutten & Kerkstra, 1996). The EURHOMAP (Mapping Professional Home Care in Europe) project has been developed to assess aspects of the home-care sector in 31 European countries and the results of this study are reported in this volume. Policy-makers, academics and those responsible for service delivery will find comparable descriptive information on many aspects of the organization, financing and provision of home care across Europe. Formal structures are addressed as well as the reality of home care, including system failures and unmet needs.

In this book, 'home care' refers primarily to services provided by professionals in the homes of adult recipients, but informal care and the role of non-professionals in home care have not been left aside. The text will note explicitly any reference to informal care. Likewise, the focus is not only on regulation for professionally provided home care but also on regulation aiming at stimulating informal care. The latter is likely to become increasingly important.

Home care has a different meaning and purpose across countries, varying from a safety net for those without relatives to a right for all citizens. Consequently, countries currently show strong differences in features such as the role of professionals in home care; citizens' eligibility for services; financial

---
1 See: http://ec.europa.eu/health/programme/key_documents/index_en.htm#anchor3.

conditions; and regulatory mechanisms that steer the sector. Different historical developments have largely influenced these policy differences (Burau, Theobald & Blank, 2007). With its focus on 'regulated' home care, this book provides more comprehensive coverage of home care as it is found in countries with well developed home-care sectors.

This volume is structured as follows. This first chapter provides an introduction to home care in its context, including social services and health-care systems as well as demographic developments. This is followed by definitions, the conceptual framework and methods used in the study. Chapter 1 also describes what was known on home-care from the literature and what this study has added to this knowledge. Chapter 2 will describe the choices European countries have made on home-care related policies, including governmental responsibilities for home care; the coherence of visions and regulation; how access to services is controlled and its quality assurance regulated. The chapter also describes prevailing funding mechanisms and how service providers are paid. Chapter 3 focuses on clients in the context of the home-care sector, in particular on eligibility and aspects of accessibility to formal services, affordability and the role of informal caregivers. Chapter 4 explores differences in the management of the care process, including coordination between different types of services, competition among providers and maintenance of the quality of services at the operational level. The fifth and final chapter draws conclusions and looks ahead by considering the home-care related challenges raised throughout the book and the responses that have been identified.

Volume II (online at www.nivel.eu/eurhomap) contains structured descriptions of the home-care sector in each of the 31 countries studied.

1.2 Challenges of home care in Europe

Given a choice between care in an institution or at home, most people would prefer to stay in their own home (TNS Opinion & Social, 2007). This may be a major argument for the legitimacy of care provided at recipients' homes but it is not the only one. The provision of services in patients' homes is typically more cost-effective than in institutions, particularly if available informal care is used effectively (Tarricone & Tsouros, 2008). Expectations about the possibilities for home care have grown as new technology facilitates care coordination and enables distant monitoring and more complex treatments in the home situation (Tarricone & Tsouros, 2008). In many countries, the balance of long-term care tends to shift towards home-based care, as many governments pursue the concept of 'ageing in place' (OECD, 2005).

In addition to these specific arguments, general arguments applicable to long-term care are also valid for home care. Health and social care systems are facing growing demand as a consequence of demographic and societal developments in most European countries (OECD, 2011). In the EU-27 at present, for every person over the age of 65 there are four people of working age, but by 2050 there will be only two. As a consequence, demand for long-term care, including home care, can be expected to increase in the decades to come. If certain types of home-care services would indeed prove more cost-effective than institutional care, demand for home care could grow faster as a result of substitution policies.

Governments' current role in home care is not evident. On the one hand, they are under pressure to anticipate the future by developing at least a vision on home care and taking appropriate steering measures. On the other hand, the health and social care sectors in some countries are showing a trend of retreating governments that are giving more space to private initiatives. In public opinion, however, government has a clear role in the provision of care. Europeans generally (90% or more) hold the opinion that home care and institutional care for elderly people should be provided by public authorities (TNS Opinion & Social, 2007). Concerning financial implications, less than half (48%) think that children should be financially liable for the care of their elderly parents if their parents' income is not sufficient (TNS Opinion & Social, 2007). Although professional care is clearly preferred, only 34% believe that care services for dependent people in their own homes is affordable (TNS Opinion & Social, 2007). Public opinions about the first choice for help with a dependent parent and the affordability of home care vary strongly between European countries (see Fig. 1.1).

One important question is the extent to which the expectations of European citizens regarding publicly financed care can be sustained in the future and whether the relatively generous home-care schemes that exist in a number of countries will be sustainable in the light of the continuing economic downturn. In countries where home care has been decentralized, financial pressure in the sector may generate geographical differences and thus become a challenge to equity (Burau, Theobald & Blank, 2007).

In addition to the expected growing demand and financial constraints in the home-care sector, the availability of home-care workers is another possible challenge. Home care is labour intensive and the question is whether sufficient qualified staff will be available if the ratio between the working age population and the elderly population changes as mentioned above. Scarcity also applies to informal carers, such as spouses, children, other relatives and volunteers. In many countries informal care is becoming scarcer as a result of growing mobility, urbanization and women's increasing participation in the labour

Fig. 1.1 *Preference for professional home care and opinion on affordability of home care*

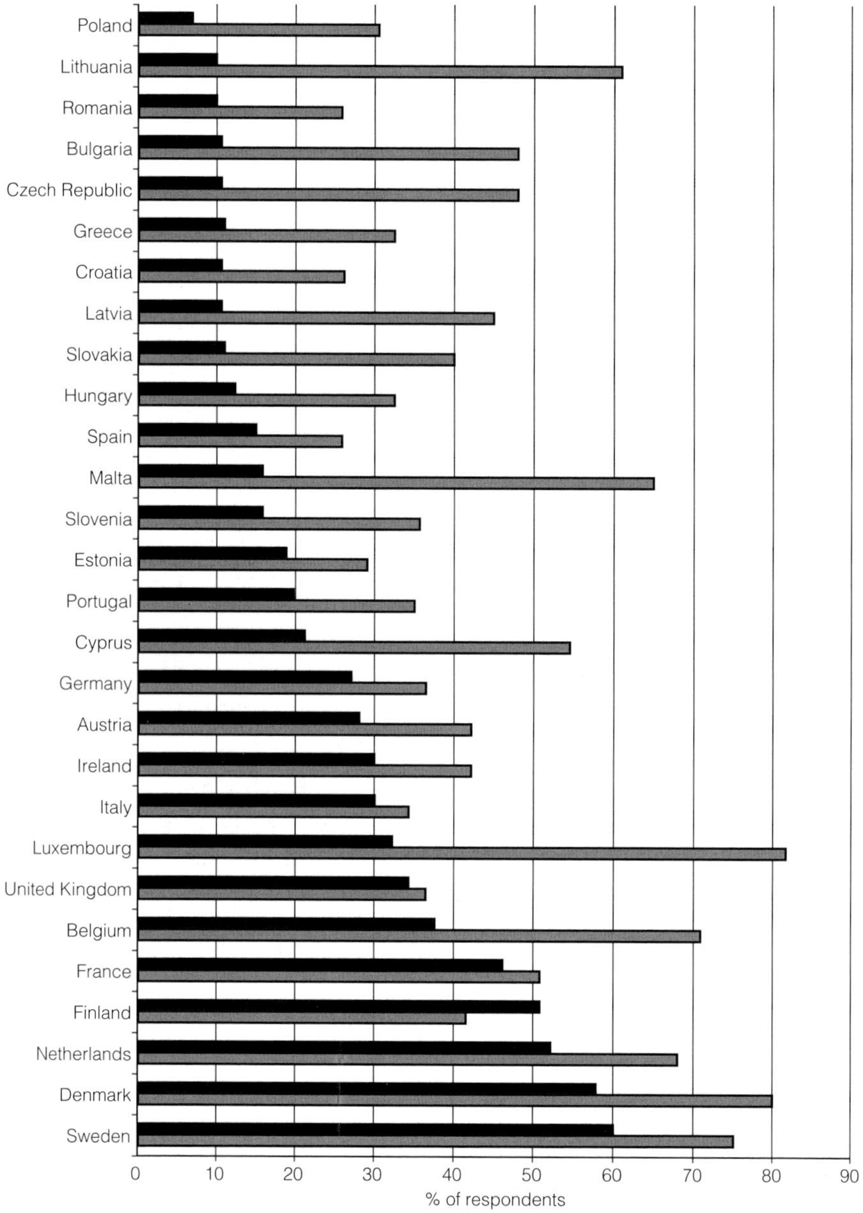

■ Public or private service providers should visit their home and provide them with appropriate help[a]
■ % of respondents having an opinion on the affordability of home care, agreeing that professional care at home is available at an affordable cost[b]

[a] Data based on the question: *"Imagine an elderly father or mother who lives alone and can no longer manage to live without regular help due to his or her physical or mental health condition. In your opinion, what would be the best option for people in this situation?"*

Possible answers: moving to a nursing home; living with one of their children; children visiting to provide care; don't know.

[b] Data based on the question *"Could you please tell me if you agree or disagree with each of the following statements regarding this issue?"*

Source: TNS Opinion & Social, 2007.

market, the latter traditionally providing the lion's share of informal care (Mestheneos & Triantafillou, 2005; Gibson, Gregory & Pandya, 2003). Conversely, the current economic crisis could have a softening effect on the workforce problem in the care sector. In times of economic stagnation and growing unemployment, working in the care sector can be perceived as a relatively safe haven.

The current turbulent situation in the European Union (EU) also affects non-EU members and so all countries are likely to be forced to reorientate their health and social care systems, including home-care services. Our study found that home care is a relatively new phenomenon in central and eastern Europe. In such countries the current financial constraints are not favourable for further development and what used to be best practices may no longer be taken automatically as models to strive for. Even countries with traditionally well developed home-care systems are likely to be forced to look for new, more sustainable models of care provision. Probably there will be a greater need than ever before for foreign experiences and models of provision to develop new forms of care that balance quality, equity and costs and contain an optimal mix of professional and volunteer-provided care.

Decision-making is extremely complex as home care is so heterogenous. It consists of care provided for the long term; for short-term recuperation after hospital discharge; and palliative care (Genet et al., 2011). Furthermore, and this distinction will be made throughout the book, it consists of both social and health care services (Burau, Theobald & Blank, 2007). The social care system is more often organized at local level, has a lower level of professionalization and is less generously funded than the health-care system (Leichsenring et al., 2005).

The home-care sector is also complex because of its interdependency with other sectors that have a role in enabling people to stay at home – for instance, the hospital sector, primary health care, housing and the social welfare sector. Coordination is essential, not just between professional care providers but also between professionals and informal caregivers (Bonsang, 2009).

1.2.1 Differences in the urgency and severity of challenges

The urgency and severity of challenges may vary between countries as there are not only great differences in national wealth but also in the indicators of future demand for care. In 2010 the purchasing power per inhabitant differed by a factor of six between Luxembourg and Bulgaria (Eurostat, 28-06-2011).[2] Similarly, there are marked variations in expenditures on long-term

---

2 Eurostat [online/offline database]. Luxembourg, European Commission (http://epp.eurostat.ec.europa.eu/portal/page/portal/statistics/themes, accessed 6 June 2012).

care – in eight Organisation for Economic Co-operation and Development (OECD) countries in 2008 these varied from less than 0.5% to about 3.6% of gross domestic product (GDP) (OECD, 2010). Also, the allocation of these expenditures to nursing and social services differed between countries. A more relevant indicator for the target population for home care is older people's ability to pay for services they need. This shows extreme differences between countries. On average, 22% of the EU-27 population over 65 years old is at risk of social exclusion or poverty (Eurostat, 15-02-2011). Bulgaria (66%), Latvia (55.5%) and Cyprus (50.1%) are far above this average. The risk of social exclusion and poverty is lowest in Luxembourg (6.2%), the Netherlands (8.1%) and the Czech Republic (11.7%) (Eurostat, 15-02-2011). Clearly, elderly people in these latter countries will be in better positions to cope with measures of increased private payments for services.

The balance between the working population and the retired population indicates the burden of elderly care on the working population. Until 2050, the proportion of the population aged over 65 years will increase in comparison to the population aged between 15 and 64 years. The old-age dependency ratio differs widely across countries (see Fig. 1.2). In countries with a high old-age dependency ratio, relatively fewer people will be available to pay for and care for their elderly people. In 2050, the old-age dependency ratio is expected to be relatively high in Slovenia, Italy and Spain and relatively low in Cyprus, Luxembourg and the United Kingdom (see Fig. 1.2). Between 2010 and 2050 the increase in this dependency ratio will be most drastic in Ireland, Malta, Slovakia and Poland.

A specific indicator for demand in the shorter term is the self-perceived severe limitations in daily activities among the elderly population. These also vary between countries, though to a lower degree (see Fig. 1.3). Some of the highest proportions of the elderly population with severe perceived limitations are found in Portugal, Slovakia and Greece; the lowest are found in Malta, the Netherlands and Switzerland. In countries where more elderly people perceive limitations the need for (professional and/or informal) care may be expected to be higher.

It may be concluded that a number of (externally caused) challenges that policy-makers are facing in the home-care sector have similar features across Europe. However, they are addressed in quite different national situations.

Fig. 1.2 Old-age dependency ratio in Europe, 2010 and 2050

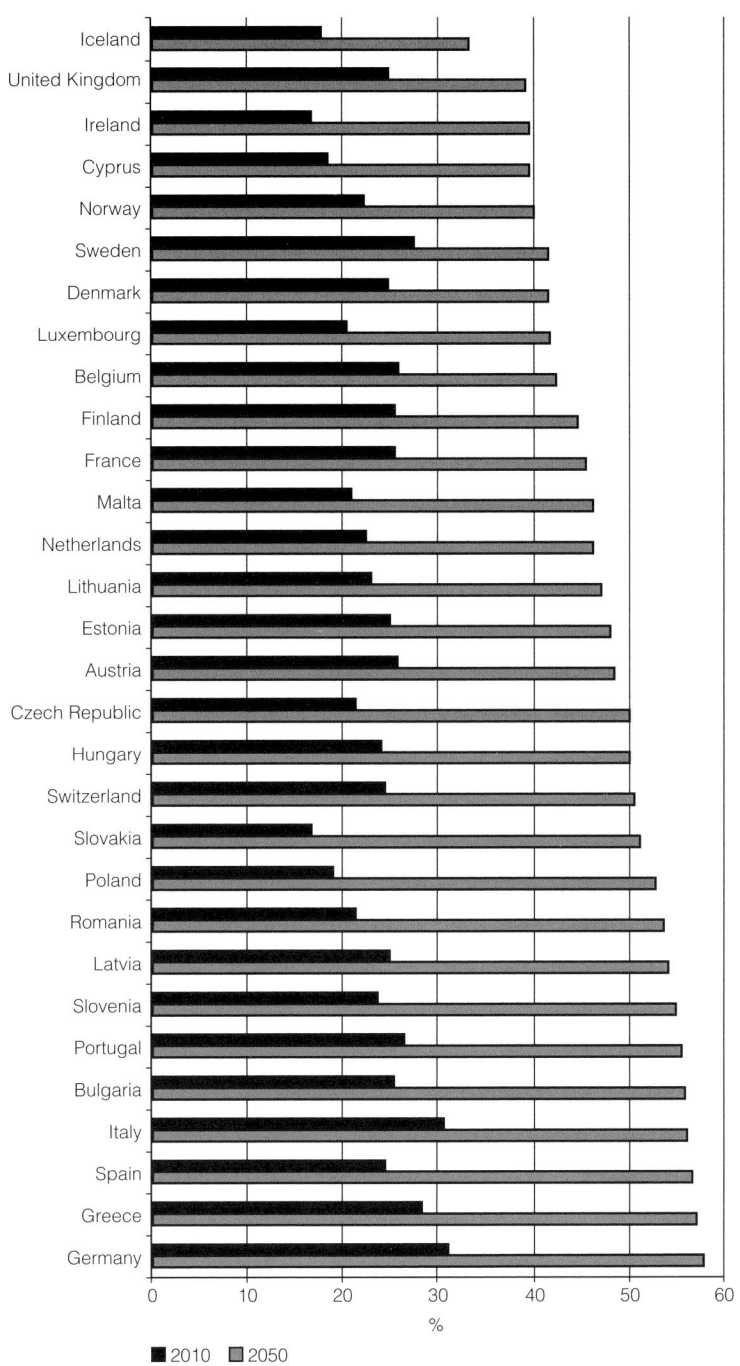

Note: The old-age dependency ratio is the projected number of people aged 65 and over expressed as a percentage of the projected number of people aged between 15 and 64 (Eurostat, last updated: 17–06–2011).

Fig. 1.3 *Self-perceived limitations in daily activities[a] of retired people in Europe*

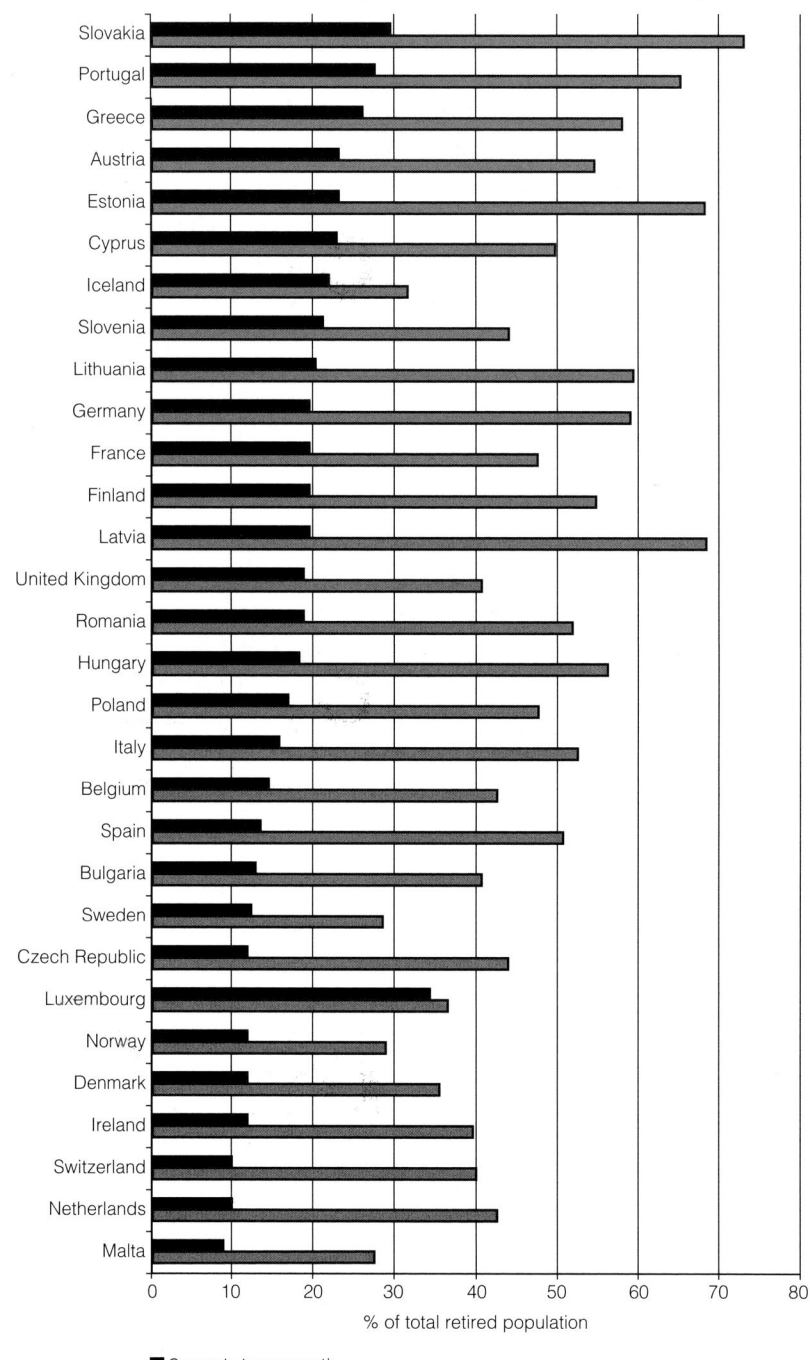

■ Severely hampered[b]
▨ Hampered to some extent[c]

[a] Restriction of activity for at least the past 6 months – in 2009; [b] Limited due to health problems, but not strongly; [c] Strongly limited due to health problems

Source: Eurostat, last updated 22-02-2011.

1.3 Definition of home care

This study showed that the term 'home care' is understood very differently across countries and sectors. The services included vary considerably among countries and even 'home' turns out to be an elastic term. Many studies on home care lack precision in defining the activities, goals and even the target groups of home care (Thomé, Dykes & Hallberg, 2003; Breedveld, 2004). Home care can be conceived of as any care provided behind someone's front door or, more generally, referring to services enabling people to stay living in their home environment. In some countries, 'someone's front door' can include a home for the elderly. As regards the type of services, home care may refer to care given only by professionals or in combination with care given by a spouse or relative (personal care or housekeeping).

The EURHOMAP study has defined home care as care provided by professional carers within clients' own homes. Professional care that relieves informal caregivers (respite care) has also been taken into account. The study has been limited to care provided to adults. Furthermore, home care has been considered in its context, such as demographic developments and attitudes in society towards informal care. Although the main focus is on formal care (provided by professional carers), informal care has been taken into account as complementary to formal care and as a codeterminant in the allocation of formal care. Informal care is provided by spouses or family members, friends and volunteers who are usually not paid; and by privately hired non-professionals who are paid informally.

The definition of home care used in this book includes not only long-term care (as in the OECD definition), but also short-term care provided at home. The scope of home-care services can be preventive, acute, rehabilitative or palliative in kind (OECD, 2005). As demand is becoming increasingly complex, mixed types of home care (social-care services as well as health-care services) are becoming more prevalent. The type and range of services included in our study are social services – such as domestic aid, personal care and technical aid – as well as nursing services (Hutten & Kerkstra, 1996; Burau, Theobald & Blank, 2007). Hence, this book does not deal exclusively with care for frail elderly people, it also includes patients in need of home care after hospitalization and adults with disabilities.

Some types of care mentioned may need clarification. Domestic-aid services relate to instrumental activities of daily living (IADL), such as using the telephone, shopping, food preparation, housekeeping, transportation, taking medication and financial administration (Lawton & Brody, 1969). Personal-care services provide assistance with dressing, feeding, washing and toileting, and getting in or out of bed (also called personal activities of daily living). The provision of health information and education is known as supportive nursing services. Technical nursing includes activities such as assistance putting on prostheses or elastic stockings; changing stomas and urinal bags; help with bladder catheters; skin care; disinfection and prevention of bedsores; oxygen administration; catheterization and giving intravenous injections. Rehabilitative nursing refers to occupational therapy or physiotherapy. This book also differentiates between social care and health care provided at home. The labelling of services as either social care or health care depends on the characteristics and boundaries of both systems in a country – home nursing is normally part of the health-care system; domestic aid is part of social services. The position of personal care varies. This is an important distinction since home health care and social home care are usually regulated differently.

Informal care (e.g. provided by spouse, relatives or friends) and formal home care (professionally provided) are less distinct than they may seem. The availability of informal care often may make the difference between a patient or client staying at home or being institutionalized. The boundary between informal and formal care is even more blurred when informal caregivers receive formal payments, for instance in the context of personal budget schemes.

1.4 Conceptual framework

For the EURHOMAP study, the conceptual framework of Murray and Frenk (2000) was taken as the basis on which we added new elements. Murray and Frenk identified the following functions of a system: financing, stewardship, service delivery, and generating (human and physical) resources. *Financing* was understood as: *the process by which revenue is collected from primary and secondary sources, accumulated in fund pools and allocated to provider priorities. Stewardship* was defined as: *setting, implementation and monitoring of the rules for the … system; assuring a level playing field for all actors in the system … ; and defining strategic directions for the … system as a whole.* Finally, the *delivery of services* was defined as: *the combination of inputs into a production process that takes place in a particular organizational setting and that leads to the delivery of a series of interventions* (Murray & Frenk, 2000).

Murray and Frenk's concept of 'stewardship' has been substituted by the more neutral and broader term 'governance'. This refers to policy development, supervision of home-care systems and regulation to steer it where necessary. As home care consists of health care and social services, which are usually not well integrated, governance often has a divided nature. For this reason, different governmental levels will need to be considered.

Financing is a vital function in the framework. First, it implies the collection of funds (e.g. via insurance, taxation or private payment). Secondly, it refers to fund pooling which aims to reduce the individual risks of citizens through insurance schemes. Thirdly, purchasing is the spending of funds to cover the costs of home-care services. Like the governance function, financing can be split into health care and social services and includes components at governmental levels (Murray & Frenk, 2000; Kutzin, Jakab & Cashin, 2010).

Resource generation is another essential system function. This study's framework (see Fig. 1.4) focuses on 'human resources' as home care is extremely labour intensive and physical resources are relatively less dominant. The availability of sufficient staff with adequate qualifications and skills to respond to the needs for home care in the population is particularly important. This includes professional development, training and continuing education.

The *service delivery* function identified in the framework encompasses the activities organized within publicly and privately owned agencies and institutions which deliver social and health-care services in the clients' homes. Care coordination, which includes the monitoring of clients' needs, has been given its own place in the box 'service provision'. The fragmented character of the concept that is home care, and the absence of an institutional setting of service delivery, make coordination in home care more challenging than elsewhere. Integrated care or seamless care is the result of coordination.

In addition to the elements identified by Murray and Frenk, this study also discerns the function of safeguarding the quality of services. This is a particular challenge in home care due to its fragmented nature and the difficulty of controlling situations in the homes of clients. Another two elements have been added to the Murray and Frenk framework – (i) the procedure required to apply for care; and (ii) the assessment of clients' needs. These have an independent place in our framework. Assessment and application for care are not always made by those who actually provide the services. Hence, it is crucial to distinguish this process from the delivery process in order to understand differences between countries. Allocated on the basis of a needs assessment, services (nursing, social or other) are then delivered by (public or privately owned) service providers.

The three levels of the home-care system that can be distinguished in this framework will also serve as the organizing thread throughout the rest of this book – (i) policy; (ii) the clients or recipients of care; and (iii) the management of the care process as delivered by care providers. The policy perspective concerns issues of funding and regulating home care; the clients' perspective relates to issues of access to the home-care system and the client system (which includes the informal caregivers); the management perspective refers to the delivery of care, quality assurance and human resource management. The heart of the framework as depicted in Fig. 1.4 is the client and his or her informal caregivers. An application for a needs assessment is submitted either from the client system or directly from a residential setting (e.g. hospital or nursing home).

The financing system consists of the remuneration of providers and can be either based on budgets or related to services allocated to clients. In addition, clients can be eligible for direct payments to purchase care, for instance through personal budgets or voucher systems. The framework also shows a financial flow from clients to the system, usually in the form of (co)payments.

Fig. 1.4 *Conceptual framework*

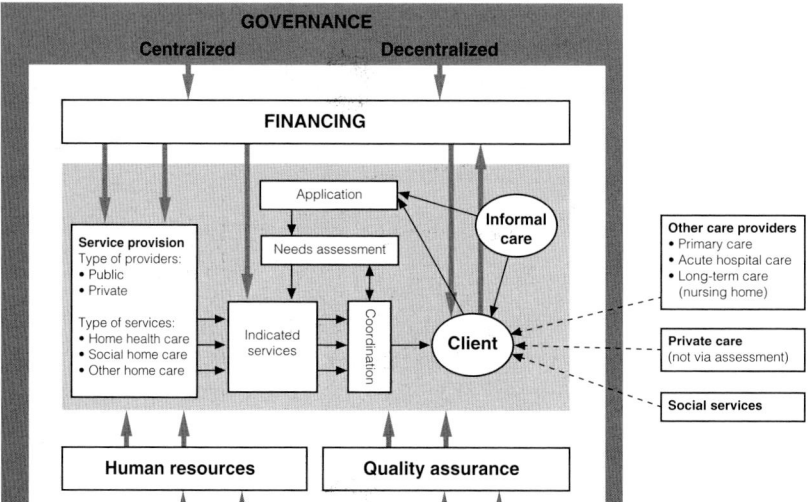

Obviously, home-care services do not function in a vacuum and there are many external influences. Some 'nearby' influences from the health-care system, social services and the privately financed market for home care have been depicted in the figure. The EURHOMAP study has taken many of these and other contextual aspects into account because they enhance the understanding of differences in home-care systems in Europe. The scheme in Fig. 1.4 is designed to explain functions and to clarify their interrelations and influences, indicated with arrows. The figure does not take the historical development of home care in countries into account.

1.5 Problem and research questions

The 2006 Public Health Work Plan of the European Commission pointed to an information gap on home care in Europe. This study aims to fill this gap by describing the formal home-care systems in 31 countries (27 EU countries, Croatia, Iceland, Norway and Switzerland).

The study addressed three research questions:

1. What does the scientific literature reveal about home care in Europe?

2. What home-care services are available in European countries; how are they financed; how do people have access to these services; how is service delivery organized; what is the role of informal caregivers?

3. What are the current trends and challenges in the home-care sector in European countries?

These questions are answered in this book, on a web site (www.nivel.eu/eurhomap) and by articles in scientific journals.

1.6 Methods

1.6.1 Systematic literature review

The study began with an exploration of the current knowledge on home care in Europe and the gaps therein. Scientific literature about home care in one or more of the 31 countries was studied systematically (Genet et al., 2011). In addition, an inventory was compiled on the focus and conclusions of comparative international projects on home care and related areas.

1.6.2 Instruments for comparison

The EURHOMAP study has used two instruments to describe and compare home care across Europe:

1. A *comprehensive set of indicators* which served as the structured framework for data collection in each country. These were developed on the basis of the systematic literature review and the expertise of partners in the project consortium.

2. *Four case narratives (vignettes)* with related questionnaires. Developed within the consortium, the vignettes described different situations of people living at home and in need of various sorts of care. Questions related to the vignettes asked about the application procedure, eligibility for home care, which services were available, financial implications, the role of informal caregivers and the alternatives if home care was not an option.

In each country, experts familiar with the daily practice of home care in their country have answered these vignettes, providing a more integrated and 'client-centred' picture of home care.

1.6.3 Data gathering

The study used both desk research and interviews with country experts to gather the information needed. Experts were interviewed to complete or verify the information gained from initial desk research. These interviews formed the basis of further desk research. The sources used for the desk research are listed below.

- *Systematic search of the scientific literature.* This was undertaken as a first step to disclose available knowledge about home care in Europe. Results have been summarized in section 1.7.
- *Study of international and national statistical sources.* For reasons of comparability, it was preferred to use data from international sources such as the OECD Health Data, the WHO Health for All database and Eurostat.
- *Study of policy documents and research reports/articles* in each country and on a European level (e.g. through projects such as SHARE[3] and Eurofamcare[4]). Most national documents have been accessed via local experts.

Around ten experts per country have been consulted, either for answering questions on case narratives or for providing information on the indicators. The experts were policy-makers, managers of home-care agencies and coordinators in home-care related organizations (such as needs assessment agencies; insurers). Data were collected until 2009 with a few exceptions. Where data refer to later years, this is noted in the text.

1.6.4 Data analysis

The project consortium set out to develop uniformly structured descriptions of home care in each country, to produce comparative overviews and to synthesize the results. Partners in the consortium analysed the information on each of the countries for which they were responsible. A uniform format was used to produce the country reports presented in Volume II and on the web site (www.nivel.eu/eurhomap).

1.6.5 A note on the comparability of results

Although the domain of home care was clearly defined and the collected information was critically checked, the researchers are aware that it has not

---

[3] Survey of Health, Ageing and Retirement in Europe (http://www.share-project.org/).

[4] Services for Supporting Family Carers of Elderly People in Europe: Characteristics, Coverage and Usage (http://www.uke.de/extern/eurofamcare/).

always been possible to collect information that exactly conforms to our definition from the multitude of sources used. The OECD database did not provide data on all countries involved in this study. In addition, national reports and documents as well as the experts interviewed had different views and conceptions of home care. 'Unusually' classified data underwent some transformation to make it fit the database.

It is also important to note the different reference dates of the information. The data were gathered between 2008 and 2010. In some places information was added later but this has been indicated in the text. The latest available information was used, and therefore does not always refer to the same year in each country. Furthermore, information concerning care for a part of the population or some regions of a country was sometimes used in the absence of national representative data. These limitations reflect the current state and comparability of information on home care in Europe.

In addition to these notes on the comparability of information, it is important to stress that different contexts should be taken into consideration while making comparisons. Cross-country learning requires consideration of contextual factors such as the available alternatives to home care (family care, voluntary work and institutional care options) and the financial means available. Information on the context of home care in each country has been described in the country reports in Volume II, available on the web site (www.nivel.eu/eurhomap).

1.7 What was known about home care in Europe

Conclusions from the literature review and the inventory of comparative international projects on home care and related areas are described below.

1.7.1 From international research projects: explaining differences and concern with integration of care, informal care and social exclusion

Relevant international projects related to home care have been reviewed and various comparative studies on long-term care have been identified, many funded by the EU. Trend studies are clear about the growing demand for long-term institutional as well as home care. Comparative studies point to many differences in the financing, delivery and governance of home care, or the overarching long-term care or social-care systems (e.g. OECD, 2005; Tarricone & Tsouros, 2008; Pickard et al., 2007; Billings & Leichsenring, 2005; Burau, Theobald & Blank, 2007; Nies & Berman, 2004; Blackman, Brodhurst & Convery, 2001;

Carpenter et al., 2004). Projections of long-term care expenditures showed that the southern countries especially could expect a strong increase of expenditures in the decades to come (Pickard et al., 2007). An OECD study on long-term care, expenditure, financing and recipients pointed to rising demand and a lack of coordination of services (OECD, 2005). A more recent OECD overview of the need for, and supply of, home care in European countries pointed to contrasts in home-care financing and organization, but the methods and scope of the study were not clear (Tarricone & Tsouros, 2008). A study on seven European countries looked at home-care governance by governments, the market, voluntary organizations and families. This showed that financing, delivery and rules on both formal and informal care were governed quite differently (Burau, Theobald & Blank, 2007). Governance concerning formal home care appeared to differ mainly on the dimensions of the private–public sector and national–local level. These differences were explained by differences in institutions (i.e. state support for formal care delivery and for female labour-market participation) and ideas (i.e. relatives' work and care in households). A study by Wiener, Tilly & Cuellar (2003) addressed financing and the costs of home care in three countries. This identified strengths and weaknesses of home-care programmes (including problems related to the labour force).

The development and evaluation of assessment instruments as a management tool have been practised extensively in the context of interRAI, a research network covering over 20 countries (http://www.interrai.org). The assessment system for home care developed in interRAI consists of a minimum data set and client assessment protocols designed to collect standardized information on a broad range of aspects. The perspective of care recipients was considered by the AdHOC project concerning home care for the elderly in 11 countries. Diagnoses and utilization of care were linked to settings (institutional or ambulatory) and to service characteristics. The resulting national profiles showed contrasts between northern and southern Europe in both the situation of recipients of care and the funding and provision of services (Carpenter et al., 2004). Another study examined clients' control over, and choice of, home- and community-care services. These reported examples of schemes aimed to shift the balance of control from agencies to users, including personal budgets in the Netherlands and direct payments in England (Wiener, Tilly & Cuellar, 2003).

Blackman, Brodhurst & Convery (2001) explored the diversity of social care provision for older people in six countries, using the central concept of social exclusion. Case studies clarified how the organization and delivery of care were shaped by the wider welfare state regime. The study points to the relationship between national awareness of social exclusion and the way in which services have developed. The SOCCARE[5] project identified a strong variation in models of provision and the degree of development and availability of services in five countries. Differences were related to cultural traditions and the diversity of family structures, confirming the findings of Burau, Theobald & Blank (2007). The PROCARE study in nine European countries focused on the integration of long-term care services. Large differences were found between the health- and social-care systems in these countries (Billings & Leichsenring, 2005). National parameters such as financing and organization, systemic development and professionalization were taken into account, as well as relevant societal values and political approaches. The study concluded that a European vision on integrated care for the elderly is absent and that health- and social-care systems remain poorly integrated within countries (Leichsenring & Aleszewski, 2004; Billings & Leichsenring, 2005). The CARMEN network compared methods for integrated care. Fragmentation between acute care, long-term care, social care, housing and welfare was found to be common in all countries. The project produced a European research agenda for integrated care for the elderly (Nies & Berman, 2004).

Eurofamcare reviewed the situation of family carers – informal care – in 6 (later 17) countries, taking account of available supportive services, care settings and labour market trends. This showed a need for support services for informal caregivers, including respite care; day care arrangements; specialized (palliative) care; volunteer support and technological application in the home situation (Mestheneos & Triantafillou, 2005). In an eight-country study, Viitanen (2007) found public expenditure on formal care reduced informal care. However, many studies performed on data from the SHARE international scientific database on ageing showed this relationship to be more complicated and dependent on the type of formal care and informal caregivers (e.g. Brandt, Haberkern & Szydlik, 2009; Bonsang, 2009; Bolin, Lindgren & Lundborg, 2007; Pommer, Woittiez & Stevens, 2007).

In addition to informal care, home visits made by general practitioners (GPs) also seem to be a relevant contextual factor. A study in general practice in 18 European countries provided information on GPs' role in home care (Boerma, 2003). Home visits were a regular task of GPs in most countries but the number of home visits per GP differed strongly and appeared to be related to their different roles in health-care systems. A decreasing trend was observed in GP home visits across Europe (Boerma, 2003).

Concerning specific conditions, studies on dementia care should be mentioned. An OECD study on dementia care in nine countries pointed to the complexity

---

[5] Families, Work and Social Care in Europe (http://ec.europa.eu/research/social-sciences/projects/102_en.html).

of this care and to the need to alleviate the burden on family members (Moise, Schwarzinger & Um, 2004). Alzheimer Europe, a nongovernmental organization (NGO) aiming to raise awareness about dementia, has also performed research on home care in Europe. This showed wide inter-country differences in the proportions of people with Alzheimer disease living in their own home. Furthermore, half of the informal caregivers of patients with Alzheimer disease provided more than ten hours of care per day in the later stages of the disease. Development and greater (financial) accessibility to formal home care were reported to be essential (Alzheimer Europe, 2010).

The application of technology is increasingly a subject of research since it can enhance users' independence and expand the possibilities of home care. For instance, the Ambient Assisted Living programme (AAL) addressed the use of intelligent products in the home environment and the provision of remote (care) services (Steg et al., 2006). Aspects of 'ambient assisted living' were reported from six countries.

1.7.2 From scientific literature: limited information and strong intra- and inter-country variation

A systematic review of the literature helped to build the framework presented above. This review was carried out to find out what has been reported about home care in Europe in the scientific literature (Genet et al., 2011). The search focused on English language papers published in the past decade related to 31 European countries. It was undertaken in the following databases: *CINAHL*®, the Cochrane Library, Embase, MEDLINE®, PsycINFO®, Sociological Abstracts, Social Services Abstracts and Social Care Online. The countries included were the 27 EU member states, Croatia, Iceland, Norway and Switzerland. The search identified 5133 potentially relevant studies which were assessed in three successive rounds by pairs of reviewers. The first round assessed only the title of the publication; the second round considered both title and abstract. Full texts were independently assessed in the third round. Publications had to report empirical studies about home care as defined, dealing with the topics specified and covering at least one of the 31 identified countries.

The review showed that little information on home care was available in the scientific literature. Just 74 studies could be traced, of which only a limited number had an international comparative perspective. No information was available on home care in 13 (of 31 included) countries. In general, little information was found on central and eastern European countries. One third of the studies focused on one of the identified topics only – organization and service delivery; financing; clients and informal caregivers; or policy and regulation of home care. The scale of the studies was usually small and the level of detail differed considerably. The selected articles focused on a variety of topics but most was reported about home-care clients' characteristics, the organization of services and the process of delivery.

Strong indications of large differences were found in policies, the practical organization of home-care services and the availability of home care. With regard to *policy and regulation*, several countries had developed a clear vision on home care and set criteria for eligibility, some of which take account of the financial situation and availability of informal care. Countries showed differences in the way that responsibilities for policy-making, financing and organization were distributed between central and local governments, and in whether policy on home care was integrated or segmented (i.e. separate for social care and health care).

Regarding *financing*, the articles mainly focused on funding mechanisms and underfunding. Countries differed with respect to the level and mechanisms of public funding (i.e. tax-based or insurance-based; national or regional). Usually a mix of funding mechanisms was in place. Reported problems were budget shortages, poor affordability of home care and problems related to separate funding schemes for nursing care and other types of home care. A north-south gradient seemed to exist – the north having more comprehensive publicly funded home-care systems. However, countries with relatively abundant home-care systems seemed to develop a trend to concentrate on the core clients – those with the highest needs for care.

Several articles focused on the organizations that provide home care and on the needs of the assessment procedure. A variety of *providers* was identified: public, private non-profit-making, private profit-making, or a mix of these; and their importance differed between countries. Providers could offer a range of home-care services or specialize in only one. Several countries showed a trend of increasing private provision (contracted providers). Regulation sometimes affected the traditional and the new players differently and working conditions in the private sector could differ from those in the public sector. Countries also differed in the organization (and formalization) of needs assessment. Finally, several articles concentrated on the working conditions of home-care professionals and on arrangements to increase the quality of care.

Regarding *clients and informal caregivers*, studies examined the predictors of receiving home care in a country (mainly client characteristics). Predictors, including the availability of informal caregivers, seemed to differ between countries. Possibilities to pay informal caregivers and for respite care were shown to have been available in some countries but absent in most others. Several papers reported client-centred arrangements such as cash-for-care schemes; such schemes could transfer the burden of coordination to the clients with free choice.

In some countries, access to, and the availability of, home care differed between municipalities and between the social and health sectors as a result of differences in policy, regulation, modes of delivery and financing schemes. Several countries had decentralized home care, allowing lower-level authorities the possibility to set priorities and develop their own conditions and criteria. This may give rise to inequalities in access to, and the quality of, services between regions or municipalities. Mechanisms to safeguard the fair allocation and integrated provision of home-care services were reported but, at the same time, coordination and integration were reported to be problematic in several countries.

1.8 What this book adds to the current knowledge

The literature search allows two conclusions to be drawn. First, there is little recent comparative information specifically related to home-care financing, organization and coherence of service provision in the EU. Many studies have a general focus on either social care or long-term care. Secondly, most studies disclose large international variation, but provide little insight or understanding of the extent to which differences are related to characteristics of the broader care systems, especially the health-care context in the countries.

The EURHOMAP project provides a comprehensive overview of social and health services provided at home, including short-term and long-term care, and in both regulated formal contexts and informally. It has a more comprehensive coverage of countries, using a standardized set of indicators. This will enable better comparisons and make more evidence available on the causes of differences and the possible consequences of models of financing, governance, human resources and service delivery.

Based on the broad evidence base of our study, this book offers food for thought on ways to handle the challenges facing decision-makers in Europe – some largely similar across countries, others specific to the home-care sector in a particular country. The diversity in home care in Europe is displayed through international comparisons of home-care policy and regulation; financing; the availability of home-care services from the clients' perspective; and the management of resources and services. Furthermore, results are synthesized in the light of identified problems in the home-care sector in the 31 countries. Problems tackled in one country can provide valuable lessons for others. The 31 country descriptions provided in Volume II (online only) and on the web site (www.nivel.eu/eurhomap) contain comprehensive descriptive reports on the cultural and health-care context; policy and regulation; financing;

organization and delivery; clients and informal caregivers; and current concerns and developments.

References

Alzheimer Europe (2010). *Second AE survey confirms the role of carers and the lack of adequate support.* Luxembourg (http://www.alzheimer-europe.org/index.php/EN/Policy-in-Practice2/Country-comparisons/Home-care#fragment-11, accessed 7 June 2012).

Billings J, Leichsenring K, eds. (2005). *Integrating health and social care services for older people: evidence from nine European countries.* Aldershot, Ashgate Publishing Limited (Public Policy and Social Welfare Series, Vol. 31).

Blackman T, Brodhurst S, Convery J, eds. (2001). *Social care and social exclusion: a comparative study of older people's care in Europe.* London, Palgrave Macmillan.

Boerma WGW (2003). *Profiles of general practice in Europe: an international study of variation in the tasks of general practitioners.* Utrecht, Netherlands Institute for Health Services Research.

Bolin K, Lindgren B, Lundborg P (2007). Informal and formal care among single-living elderly in Europe. *Health Economics* 17(3):393–409.

Bonsang E (2009). Does informal care from children to their elderly parents substitute for formal care in Europe? *Journal of Health Economics* 28(1):143–154.

Brandt M, Haberkern K, Szydlik M (2009). Intergenerational help and care in Europe. *European Sociological Review*, 2009, 25(5):585–601.

Breedveld E (2004). *Thuiszorg in bedrijf.* [Home care in business] [Doctoral thesis]. Tilburg, IVA Tilburg.

Burau V, Theobald H, Blank R (2007). *Governing home care: a cross national comparison.* Cheltenham, Edward Elgar Publishing.

Carpenter I et al. (2004). Community care in Europe. The Aged in Home Care project (AdHOC). *Aging Clinical and Experimental Research*, 16(4):259–269.

Eurostat [online/offline database]. Luxembourg, European Commission (http://epp.eurostat.ec.europa.eu/portal/page/portal/statistics/themes, accessed 6 June 2012).

Genet N et al. (2011). Home care in Europe: a systematic literature review. *BMC Health Services Research*, 11:207.

Gibson MJ, Gregory SR, Pandya SM (2003). *Long-term care in developed nations: a brief overview*. Washington, DC, The AARP Public Policy Institute.

Hutten JBF, Kerkstra A (1996). *Home care in Europe: a country-specific guide to its organization and financing*. Aldershot, Ashgate.

Kutzin J, Jakab M, Cashin C (2010). Lessons from health financing reform in central and eastern Europe and the former Soviet Union. *Health Economics, Policy and Law*, 5(02):135–147.

Lawton MP, Brody EM (1969). Assessment of older people: self-maintaining and instrumental activities of daily living. *Gerontologist*, 9(3):179–186.

Leichsenring K, Aleszewski AM, eds. (2004). *Providing integrated health and social care for older people: a European overview of issues at stake*. Aldershot, Ashgate.

Leichsenring K et al. (2005). Introduction: moments of truth. An overview of pathways to integration and better quality in long-term care. In: Billings J, Leichsenring K, eds. *Integrating health and social care services for older people: evidence from nine European countries*. Aldershot, Ashgate Publishing Limited:13–38.

Mestheneos E, Triantafillou J, on behalf of the EUROFAMCARE group (2005). *Supporting family carers of older people in Europe – the pan-European background*. Hamburg, University of Hamburg.

Moise P, Schwarzinger M, Um M-Y (2004). *Dementia care in 9 OECD countries: a comparative analysis*. Paris, Organisation for Economic Co-operation and Development (OECD Health Working Papers No. 13).

Murray CJ, Frenk J (2000). A framework for assessing the performance of health systems. *Bulletin of the World Health Organization*, 78(6):717–731.

Nies H, Berman P, eds. (2004). *Integrating services for older people: a resource book for managers*. Dublin, European Health Management Association.

OECD (2005). *Long-term care for older people*. Paris, Organisation for Economic Co-operation and Development.

OECD (2010). OECD Health Data [online/offline database]. *Services of long-term nursing care*. Paris, Organisation for Economic Co-operation and Development (http://www.oecd.org/health/, accessed 8 June 2010).

OECD (2011). *Help wanted? Providing and paying for long-term care*. Paris, Organisation for Economic Co-operation and Development.

Pickard L et al. (2007). Modelling an entitlement to long-term care services for older people in Europe: projections for long-term care expenditure to 2050. *Journal of European Social Policy*, 17(1):33–48.

Pommer W, Woittiez I, Stevens J (2007). *Comparing care. The care of the elderly in ten EU-countries*. The Hague, The Netherlands Institute for Social Research/SCP.

Steg H et al. (2006). *Europe is facing a demographic challenge. Ambient Assisted Living offers solutions.* Berlin, Ambient Assisted Living (http://www.aal-europe.eu/Published/reports-etc/Final%20Version.pdf, accessed 5 June 2012) (Report VDI-VDE-IT).

Tarricone R, Tsouros A, eds. (2008). *Home care in Europe: the solid facts.* Copenhagen, WHO Regional Office for Europe.

Thomé B, Dykes A-K, Hallberg IR (2003). Home care with regard to definition, care recipients, content and outcome: systematic literature review. *Journal of Clinical Nursing*, 12(6):860–872.

TNS Opinion & Social (2007). Health and long-term care in the European Union. Brussels, European Commission, *Special Eurobarometer 283/Wave 67.3*.

Viitanen T (2007). *Informal and formal care in Europe.* Sheffield. University of Sheffield and IZA (Discussion paper No. 2648).

Wiener JM, Tilly J, Cuellar AE (2003). *Consumer-directed home care in the Netherlands, England and Germany*. Washington, DC, AARP (http://assets.aarp.org/rgcenter/health/_2003_12_eu_cd.pdf, accessed 5 September 2012).

Chapter 2
The policy perspective

Nadine Genet, Madelon Kroneman, Carlos Chiatti, László Gulácsi, Wienke Boerma

2.1 Policy challenges in the European home-care sector

This chapter will discuss the policy choices made in the European home-care sector. As pointed out in the introduction, difficult choices lie ahead for those responsible for home-care systems. Policy-makers have to balance policy goals (e.g. achieving universal access, good quality of care and efficiency) and resources for different care (formal and informal, social and health, palliative, long-term and short-term). In a time of financial pressures, more efficient policy tools and division of responsibilities may be needed. Responsibilities for long-term care are already being reconsidered across Europe (Bettio & Plantenga, 2004). For instance, the different responsibilities of the private and public sector; the social-care and the health-care sector; and the related governmental levels and ministries.

Responsibilities for home care may vary from centralized (at national level) to decentralized (at municipal or regional level) and within one country may be different for home health care and home social care. Proponents of decentralized decision-making argue that it should lead to greater efficiency, a more tailored approach and thus to more appropriate home care for the individual. Opponents associate decentralization with inequality between areas. Saltman, Bankauskaite and Vrangbaek (2007) find little conclusive evidence of its effects. Still, in some studies, decentralization is shown to be associated with more innovation, more local accountability, cost-conscious behaviour but greater inequality (Saltman, Bankauskaite & Vrangbaek, 2007). In integrated care, home health care and social home care are coordinated without overlaps or gaps, therefore coordination of policies from these different sectors is increasingly important. Besides, home care should be coordinated with other care sectors, such as primary care, hospital care and long-term institutional care. Coordination of these systems has become an important policy issue with regard to long-term care (Billings & Leichsenring, 2005).

Financing, safeguarding the quality of services and equity in access to home-care services are key issues in the governance of home care. As welfare levels have risen, so have the expectations about the quality of care. However, maintaining or enhancing high levels of quality and equity in access may be challenging in a time of diminishing human and financial resources. In this context, human resources refers to both formal home-care workers and informal caregivers. Female participation in the labour force has increased all over Europe so the supply of informal carers may become more problematic (Colombo et al., 2011; Viitanen, 2007).

The complexity of decision-making in home care can be illustrated through the example of home-care financing. Decisions need to be made regarding means testing, sources of financing (i.e. private insurance, compulsory insurance, taxation, user contributions, or a combination of these), the way funds are allocated to home-care providers and, related to this, coordination of different funding streams. Different assumptions can lead to the choice of similar financing resources. For instance, the implementation of out-of-pocket payments may be based on the assumption that they discourage unnecessary or excessive use of services, but they can also be used for raising additional revenue (Mossialos et al., 2002). The choice for public financing of home care may be based on the notion that it is difficult to assess the risk and thus the amount of private income to be allocated to future home-care needs (RVZ, 2005). Furthermore, some people will not be able to afford the care they need and hence equity in access problems may arise. Hence, some form of public financing is available in all countries.

Public financing is considered to have a positive effect on equity (RVZ, 2005) and to provide stable conditions for formal care services (Burau, Theobald & Blank, 2007). However, negative effects (such as overuse) need to be addressed by implementing client co-payments or strict eligibility criteria, for instance. The organization of public financing can vary between countries. Broadly, two systems are available for public financing of home care – (i) an insurance system; or (ii) a tax-based system. Each has risks and advantages. Insurance systems can be used to pool risks; this may be done on a voluntary basis but it carries the risk of market failure. Insurance companies may exclude people with a high risk of needing their funds. Regulation such as obligatory insurance and cross subsidies (for insurance companies with high-risk patients) to spread risks may reduce the risk of market failure. A tax-based system has the advantage of being able to draw on a broad revenue base that allows trade-offs between health care and other public expenditures, as there are usually several tax mechanisms. However, this also means that the home-care budget is not earmarked and thus home care will have to 'compete' with other social needs. This could create less stable conditions for home-care providers. All these financing and regulatory choices have many more negative consequences than those presented here. This short discussion is intended to give the reader a feel for the complex interconnected issues that policy-makers are facing.

In this chapter the following aspects of policy choices across Europe will be discussed – whether governments have made explicit choices regarding home care (orientation towards home care); how responsibilities for policy decisions for the different home-care systems are divided over different levels of government; government choices about the provision of home care, access to home care, quality of care and (in section 2.3) the organization of financing. Finally (section 2.4), the trends and future challenges in these policy choices will be discussed.

2.2 Governance by European governments

This section will focus on governance of home care by governments. 'Governance' is the *process whereby elements in society wield power and authority, and influence and enact policies and decisions concerning public life ...* (Governance Working Group of the International Institute of Administrative Sciences, 1996). Governance is a broader notion than government as it involves interaction between these formal institutions and those of civil society. Governance elements addressed in this chapter concern the orientation towards home care, political decentralization, the integration of home-care services and the roles of the government inside countries.

2.2.1 Orientation of governmental visions towards home care

In most EU countries, the central government has laid down its vision on home care (see Table 2.3). Visions are the ideas of the position and shape of home care within the wider societal context, now and in the future. Visions included in this study are published by national governments in official policy documents.

National governments' visions on home care are usually formulated rather generally and do not define key concepts or specify measurable targets. Mostly, home care is discussed within the framework of long-term care[1] or policies for the elderly[2] in general. Visions usually encompass only one part of home-care

---
1 In Austria, Germany, Ireland, Luxembourg, Netherlands, Norway and Portugal.
2 In France, Romania, Slovenia and Sweden.

services – either home health care or social home care. Some countries (e.g. Czech Republic and Slovenia) have a vision for only one type and some eastern European countries have not laid down any explicit vision on home care. The absence of a detailed vision at central level is likely a result of the high level of decentralization in the home-care sector. Municipalities often define their own visions; in some countries (e.g. Finland and the Netherlands) it is their explicit responsibility to do so.

Although visions formulated by central governments differ widely across Europe, some commonalities can be found. These mostly foresee a growth in home care, often meant to replace residential and hospital care.[3] Some countries have quantified the targets of their home-care system – for example, 3% of Slovenia's 65+ population and 13–14% of Finland's 75+ population should receive home care. One common way of expanding the envisaged use of home care was to increase affordability for clients of home-care services (e.g. in Germany and Belgium).

Often, the visions refer to the ageing societies[4] and to users and their families' preference for home care (e.g. in England and Switzerland). Home care is 'adapted to the societal transformation' and is seen to fit the goal of increasing the quality of life. In this context, many governments promote the independence of people with disabilities. In Sweden, home care is seen as a means to facilitate an active life and to exercise influence in society and over the person's everyday life (maintaining security and independence in older age, ensuring respect and access to quality care). Many governments speak of the need for 'emancipated' or well informed clients.[5]

Support for informal caregivers seems to be interwoven with the vision on formal home care (e.g. in Belgium, Cyprus, Germany and Greece) as home care is seen as a way to facilitate informal care. The vision on home care in many eastern European countries (e.g. Bulgaria and Slovenia but also Greece) is furthermore entangled with employment policy. Some countries use this as a means to reduce unemployment, especially among women, by creating part-time jobs in home care.

Better coordination between different types of home-care services is also mentioned in several policy documents (e.g. in Belgium, England and Ireland). Ireland is pursuing the development of primary care teams and integrated home-care schemes have been developed in Portugal and Italy. In these countries, the cooperation between social and health-care workers at home is expected to prevent hospital admission.

---
3 For example, in Croatia, Finland, Germany, Italy, Latvia, Luxembourg and Slovenia.
4 For example, in England, Finland, France, Iceland, Italy, Malta and Sweden.
5 For example, in Austria, Czech Republic, England, Germany and the Netherlands.

Other issues addressed by these policy documents are: the level of quality of care (in Belgium, Cyprus, England and the Netherlands); increasing the home-care workforce (in Cyprus, England, the Netherlands and Norway); increasing the role of civil society within home care (in the Netherlands, Norway and Portugal); and home care as a means to prevent or ensure early detection of social isolation (in Greece and Italy).

2.2.2 Division of responsibilities between levels of government

Policy-making responsibilities are rather decentralized in many countries. Policy-making on home health care tends to be more centralized than social home care. The governmental level of control is most centralized in Belgium, Cyprus, France and Switzerland and most decentralized in Iceland and Italy. In Sweden, the regions have different levels of decentralization.

2.2.3 Integrated policy-making?

Integration of policy-making refers to the degree to which policy-making takes account of all aspects of home care and all groups of people that need home care. Table 2.1 provides an indication of the fragmentation of home-care policy.

Countries show differences in the way that responsibility for home care is divided between ministries. In most countries, several ministries have substantial roles in (for instance) the regulation, provision or financing of part of home care. Countries with one main responsible ministry are located mainly in north-west Europe. These ministries are either ministries of health or ministries of health (care) and social welfare. However, responsibility for financing and regulating home care may still be divided over different levels of governments in such countries. For home health care, financial and regulatory responsibility is often at state or regional level; for social home care this is often a municipal responsibility (as in England, France and the Netherlands). In Denmark, Ireland, Norway and Switzerland, and parts of Finland and Sweden, both social home care and home health care are the main responsibility of regional authorities or municipalities. In Finland, Norway and Sweden the level of integration is rather strong – that is, there is generally only one home-care scheme and one governmental unit responsible for policy-making. However, in many countries the level of integration of governance is low.

Most countries have more than one scheme to cover formal home care as defined in this study. Schemes may cover different age groups (as in Finland, France, Romania and Sweden) or different types of need such as long-term or acute care (as in Germany and Luxembourg). Personal assistance schemes are quite

Table 2.1 *Fragmentation of home-care policy*

Country	Is the governance on home care divided over more than one ministry? X=yes	Home-care schemes are divided according to:			
		Type of service: social and health services X=yes	Duration of care: long and short term X=yes	Age: different age groups of recipients X=yes	Other X=yes
Austria	X	X			
Belgium	X	X			
Bulgaria	X				X
Croatia		N/A	N/A	N/A	N/A
Cyprus	X	X			
Czech Republic	X	X			
Denmark		X	X		
England		X			
Estonia		X			
Finland				X	
France		X		X	
Germany		X			X
Greece	N/A				X
Hungary	X	X			
Iceland	X	X			
Ireland		X			
Italy	X	X			
Latvia	X	X			
Lithuania	X		X		
Luxembourg	X	X	X		
Malta		X			
Netherlands		X			
Norway		X			
Poland	X	X			
Portugal	X	X			
Romania	X	X		X	
Slovakia	X	X			
Slovenia	X	X			X
Spain	Xª	X			
Sweden				X	
Switzerland	N/A	X			

N/A: information not available; ª situation in 2009.

common in Europe.[6] These are characterized by the fact that disabled clients (or their families) can largely decide what care they receive from a personal assistant. These schemes may exist in parallel with in-kind provision of care, as in the Netherlands.

---

[6] For example, in Bulgaria, Croatia, Czech Republic, Romania, Slovakia and Slovenia but also in Estonia, Finland, France, Norway and Sweden.

2.2.4 Government roles in regulation, access and quality of care

In this section we will look at three areas of responsibility – regulation of: (i) home-care provision; (ii) access to publicly funded home-care services; and (iii) quality of care. A fourth area, financing and controlling expenditures, will be addressed in section 2.3. Table 2.2 provides an indication of the strength of governmental control at national level – the more bullets, the more control is exerted.

Involvement in home-care provision

In most countries, the government is involved in home-care provision. When governments provide home care, the main types of provider are usually municipalities or governmental agencies, such as health centres (see Table 2.2). This will be discussed further in Chapter 4.

When home care is outsourced to private providers they are often required to comply with certain government-set criteria in order to receive public financing. For instance, private providers need to be contracted by the government(al agency) for a certain number of hours, clients or care packages; or at least need to be registered and hence comply with certain minimum standards of care in many countries.[7] Contracting is more usual in home health care than in social home care. Providers may be contracted through municipal governments in Denmark, the Netherlands and Norway (for social home care); through governmental agencies in Ireland and Latvia; and through private insurance companies in Germany and the Netherlands (for home health care). In several countries (e.g. Portugal) a contract with a governmental agency is obligatory to run services. There are some noteworthy ways of contracting care providers, not all of which are covered by regulation. In Latvia small municipalities may contract larger municipalities to provide care; in the Netherlands home-care providers subcontract other care providers for the actual provision of care. In some countries (e.g. Slovenia) prices and/or quality requirements are set for all providers; in others (e.g. Finland and the Netherlands) individual negotiations decide the price or quality to be provided. Little is known about the privately funded home care that is not part of publicly financed home care – privately purchased by citizens, what appears to be an important type of home care (at least for a certain segment of users) seems to be outside the scope of governmental home-care regulation.

Regulation of access

Governments try to control the use of home care – provided by both publicly and privately owned (non-profit-making or profit-making) organizations – by

---

[7] For example, in Belgium, Bulgaria, Croatia, Czech Republic, Denmark, England, Estonia, Finland, Germany, Hungary, Ireland, Latvia, Malta, Netherlands, Norway, Poland, Portugal, Romania, Slovakia, Slovenia, Spain and Sweden.

Table 2.2 Strength of national governmental control over the home-care sector

Country	Provision of health care[a] • • • provided mainly by government • • part provided mainly by government • government does not mainly provide	Regulation of quality National criteria:[,b] • • • available • • partly available • not available	Co-payments set • • • • by national government • • • by municipal or regional government • • by national or regional social insurance • not by government and not by insurance		Regulation of access Eligibility Eligibility criteria • • • set by national government for main home-care services • • set by municipal/regional governments • not set for most services		Needs assessment Mainly performed by • • • public organizations • • mixed public and private organizations • private organizations	
			Home health care	Social home care	Home health care	Social home care	Home health care	Social home care
Austria	•	• • •	• • • •	• • •	• • •	• • •	•	•
Belgium	•	• •	• • •	• • •	• • •	• • •	•	•
Bulgaria	•	•	N/A	• • •	•	• •	•	• • •
Croatia	• • •	• •	• •	N/A	• • •	• • •	•	• • •
Cyprus	• • •	• •	• • • •	• • •	• • •	• • •	• • •	• • •
Czech Republic	•	• •	•	• • •	• • •	• • •	• • •	• • •
Denmark	• • •	• • •	• • •	• • •	• •	• •	• • •	• • •
England	• •	• • •	N/A	• • •	• • •	• •	• • •	• • •
Estonia	• •	• •	• •	•	•	• •	•	• • •
Finland	• • •	• •	• • •	• • •	• • •	• • •	• • •	• • •
France	•	• •	• • •	• • •	• • •	• • •	• • •	• • •
Germany	•	• • •	• • •	• •/•[c]	• • •	• • •	•	•
Greece	• • •	•	• • • •	• • •	• • •	• •	• • •	• • •
Hungary	• •	• •	• • • •	• • •	• • •	• •	•	• • •
Iceland	• • •	•	• •	• • •	• •	•	• •	•
Ireland	• • •	•	• • •	• • •	• • •	• • •	• • •	• • •

2.2.4 Government roles in regulation, access and quality of care

In this section we will look at three areas of responsibility – regulation of: (i) home-care provision; (ii) access to publicly funded home-care services; and (iii) quality of care. A fourth area, financing and controlling expenditures, will be addressed in section 2.3. Table 2.2 provides an indication of the strength of governmental control at national level – the more bullets, the more control is exerted.

Involvement in home-care provision

In most countries, the government is involved in home-care provision. When governments provide home care, the main types of provider are usually municipalities or governmental agencies, such as health centres (see Table 2.2). This will be discussed further in Chapter 4.

When home care is outsourced to private providers they are often required to comply with certain government-set criteria in order to receive public financing. For instance, private providers need to be contracted by the government(al agency) for a certain number of hours, clients or care packages; or at least need to be registered and hence comply with certain minimum standards of care in many countries.[7] Contracting is more usual in home health care than in social home care. Providers may be contracted through municipal governments in Denmark, the Netherlands and Norway (for social home care); through governmental agencies in Ireland and Latvia; and through private insurance companies in Germany and the Netherlands (for home health care). In several countries (e.g. Portugal) a contract with a governmental agency is obligatory to run services. There are some noteworthy ways of contracting care providers, not all of which are covered by regulation. In Latvia small municipalities may contract larger municipalities to provide care; in the Netherlands home-care providers subcontract other care providers for the actual provision of care. In some countries (e.g. Slovenia) prices and/or quality requirements are set for all providers; in others (e.g. Finland and the Netherlands) individual negotiations decide the price or quality to be provided. Little is known about the privately funded home care that is not part of publicly financed home care – privately purchased by citizens, what appears to be an important type of home care (at least for a certain segment of users) seems to be outside the scope of governmental home-care regulation.

Regulation of access

Governments try to control the use of home care – provided by both publicly and privately owned (non-profit-making or profit-making) organizations – by

---

[7] For example, in Belgium, Bulgaria, Croatia, Czech Republic, Denmark, England, Estonia, Finland, Germany, Hungary, Ireland, Latvia, Malta, Netherlands, Norway, Poland, Portugal, Romania, Slovakia, Slovenia, Spain and Sweden.

Table 2.2 Strength of national governmental control over the home-care sector

Country	Provision of health care[a]	Regulation of quality	Co-payments		Eligibility		Needs assessment	
	••• provided mainly by government •• part provided mainly by government • government does not mainly provide	National criteria:[b] ••• available •• partly available • not available	•••• by national government ••• by municipal or regional government •• by national or regional social insurance • not by government and not by insurance		Eligibility criteria ••• set by national government for main home-care services •• set by municipal/regional governments • not set for most services		Mainly performed by ••• public organizations •• mixed public and private organizations • private organizations	
			Home health care	Social home care	Home health care	Social home care	Home health care	Social home care
Austria	•	•••	•••	••	•••	•••	•	•
Belgium	•	••	••	••	•••	•••	•	•
Bulgaria	•	•	N/A	N/A	•	••	•	•••
Croatia	•••	•••	••	N/A	•••	•••	•	•••
Cyprus	•••	••	••••	••	•	•••	•••	•••
Czech Republic	•	••	•	•••	•••	•••	•••	•••
Denmark	•••	•••	•••	••	•••	•••	•••	•••
England	••	•••	N/A	••	•	•••	•••	•••
Estonia	•••	••	••	•	•••	•	•	•••
Finland	•••	•••	•••	••	•••	•••	•••	•••
France	•	••	••	•	•••	•••	•••	•••
Germany	•	•••	••	••/•[c]	•••	••	•	•
Greece	•••	•	•••	•••	•••	••	•••	•••
Hungary	••	••	•••	•••	•••	••	•	•••
Iceland	•••	•	•	•••	•	•	•••	•
Ireland	•••	•	•••	••	•••	•••	•••	•••

2.2.4 Government roles in regulation, access and quality of care

In this section we will look at three areas of responsibility – regulation of: (i) home-care provision; (ii) access to publicly funded home-care services; and (iii) quality of care. A fourth area, financing and controlling expenditures, will be addressed in section 2.3. Table 2.2 provides an indication of the strength of governmental control at national level – the more bullets, the more control is exerted.

Involvement in home-care provision

In most countries, the government is involved in home-care provision. When governments provide home care, the main types of provider are usually municipalities or governmental agencies, such as health centres (see Table 2.2). This will be discussed further in Chapter 4.

When home care is outsourced to private providers they are often required to comply with certain government-set criteria in order to receive public financing. For instance, private providers need to be contracted by the government(al agency) for a certain number of hours, clients or care packages; or at least need to be registered and hence comply with certain minimum standards of care in many countries.[7] Contracting is more usual in home health care than in social home care. Providers may be contracted through municipal governments in Denmark, the Netherlands and Norway (for social home care); through governmental agencies in Ireland and Latvia; and through private insurance companies in Germany and the Netherlands (for home health care). In several countries (e.g. Portugal) a contract with a governmental agency is obligatory to run services. There are some noteworthy ways of contracting care providers, not all of which are covered by regulation. In Latvia small municipalities may contract larger municipalities to provide care; in the Netherlands home-care providers subcontract other care providers for the actual provision of care. In some countries (e.g. Slovenia) prices and/or quality requirements are set for all providers; in others (e.g. Finland and the Netherlands) individual negotiations decide the price or quality to be provided. Little is known about the privately funded home care that is not part of publicly financed home care – privately purchased by citizens, what appears to be an important type of home care (at least for a certain segment of users) seems to be outside the scope of governmental home-care regulation.

Regulation of access

Governments try to control the use of home care – provided by both publicly and privately owned (non-profit-making or profit-making) organizations – by

---

[7] For example, in Belgium, Bulgaria, Croatia, Czech Republic, Denmark, England, Estonia, Finland, Germany, Hungary, Ireland, Latvia, Malta, Netherlands, Norway, Poland, Portugal, Romania, Slovakia, Slovenia, Spain and Sweden.

Table 2.2 Strength of national governmental control over the home-care sector

Country	Provision of health care[a] ••• provided mainly by government •• part provided mainly by government • government does not mainly provide	Regulation of quality National criteria:[b] ••• available •• partly available • not available	Co-payments set ••• by national government •• by municipal or regional government • by national or regional social insurance · not by government and not by insurance		Regulation of access — Eligibility Eligibility criteria ••• set by national government for main home-care services •• set by municipal/regional governments • not set for most services		Needs assessment Mainly performed by ••• public organizations •• mixed public and private organizations • private organizations	
			Home health care	Social home care	Home health care	Social home care	Home health care	Social home care
Austria	•	•••	•••	•••	•••	•••	•	•
Belgium	•	••	••	••	•••	•••	•	•
Bulgaria	•	•	N/A	•	•••	•	•	•••
Croatia	•••	••	••	N/A	•	•••	•	•••
Cyprus	•••	••	•••	•	•••	•••	•••	•••
Czech Republic	•	••	•••	•••	•••	•	•••	•••
Denmark	•••	•••	•••	••	•	•	•••	•••
England	••	•••	N/A	••	•••	•	•••	•••
Estonia	•••	••	••	•	•	•	•	•••
Finland	•••	•••	•••	••	•••	•••	•••	•••
France	•	••	••	••	•••	•••	•••	•
Germany	•	•••	•••	••/•[c]	•••	•••	•	•••
Greece	•••	•	•••	•••	•	•••	•••	•••
Hungary	••	••	•••	•••	•••	••	•	•••
Iceland	•••	•	•	•••	•	•	•••	•
Ireland	•••	•	•••	•••	•••	•••	•••	•••

Table 2.2 contd

Provision of health care[a]
- ••• provided mainly by government
- •• part provided mainly by government
- • government does not mainly provide

Regulation of quality — National criteria:[b]
- ••• available
- •• partly available
- • not available

Co-payments set
- •••• by national government
- ••• by municipal or regional government
- •• by national or regional social insurance
- • not by government and not by insurance

Regulation of access

Eligibility — Eligibility criteria
- ••• set by national government for main home-care services
- •• set by municipal/regional governments
- • not set for most services

Needs assessment — Mainly performed by
- ••• public organizations
- •• mixed public and private organizations
- • private organizations

Country	Provision of health care	Regulation of quality	Co-payments set Home health care	Co-payments set Social home care	Eligibility Home health care	Eligibility Social home care	Needs assessment Home health care	Needs assessment Social home care
Italy	•	•	••••	••	•••	•••	•••	•••
Latvia	••	•••	••	••	•••	•••	•	••
Lithuania	••	•••	••••	N/A	•••	•••	•	•
Luxembourg	•	•	••	•••	•••	•••	•	•••
Malta	••	•••	•	N/A	•••	N/A	•	•
Netherlands	•	•••	••••	••	•••	••	•	•
Norway	•••	•••	••••	•••	•••	•••	•	•••
Poland	••	••	•	•••	•••	••	•••	•••
Portugal	•	•••	N/A	•	•••	••	••	••
Romania	••	•	N/A	N/A	•••	••	••	••
Slovakia	••	••	••••	••	•••	•••	•	•••
Slovenia	••	••	••••	•••	•••	••	•••	•••
Spain	••	••	••	•••	•••	••	•••	•••
Sweden	•••	•••	•••	••	•	•	•••	•••
Switzerland	•	•••	•••	•	•••	•••	•	•

[a] Actual service provision. [b] Process and output quality criteria at national level – partly available indicates that only basic criteria are available or that criteria are available only on regional level or only for some home care programmes. [c] In some areas it is not set by governments or social insurance, in other areas it is set by regional social insurance. N/A: data not available.

setting strict eligibility criteria and requiring client co-payments. Furthermore, public organizations may perform the needs assessments (applying the eligibility criteria) or may have the final say about the assignment of care (as shown in Table 2.2). Formal eligibility criteria for publicly financed home-care services are available in most countries, except Iceland and (for part of home care) Bulgaria, Croatia and Estonia. National level eligibility criteria are detailed in Austria (for care money), Belgium (for home health care), France, Luxembourg and the Netherlands (for personal and nursing care). National level entitlement criteria are very loosely described in most countries, particularly for social home care, and therefore need to be set or elaborated by municipalities. This is less usual for home health care. A client co-payment is needed in most countries (see Table 2.2). Overuse of services can be prevented by making clients pay but it may also cause problems in equity as not all people will be able to pay. Where information is available, the strongest government controls over client co-payment levels are found in Greece, Hungary, Norway and Spain; the lowest are in the Czech Republic, Malta and Portugal. There is no clear difference in central government control over co-payment levels between social and health care. Still, municipalities and private health insurers often control social care co-payment levels and care insurance companies are more often involved in setting the level for home health care.

In many countries, municipalities or public agencies control the needs assessment for social home care. This is less so for home health care as needs assessment is often left to GPs or representatives of health insurance companies. Government responsibility for granting the care shows the same 'split' between home health care and social home care but, in most countries, the government plays a role in granting care. Individual needs assessment is generally not controlled by the government in those countries that have relatively detailed eligibility criteria. In such cases, they are in the hands of either providers or independent assessment agencies. The absence of governmental control over assignment of care is found in Belgium, Germany, the Netherlands (personal and nursing care) and several eastern European countries. In these countries GPs or, more frequently, the health insurance companies finally assign care.

Controlling quality of care

The concept of quality has been well defined in only a few countries. Where quality criteria are laid down, the criteria are generally vague; when explicit they are often not set on a national level. This holds especially true for home health care. Regulation on quality of care exists in most countries but control over quality is generally low. Regulation mainly regards a set of minimum organizational standards and when and how quality inspections (or external checks) take place.

Attaching quality requirements to licensing – such as employees' educational levels or about the use of aids – is also a usual way to control private providers (e.g. in Belgium, Luxembourg and Spain). Licensing is obligatory for public financing in some countries. Another use of quality requirements is found in Finland, where a private provider must be licensed in order for the recipient to apply for tax reductions for his/her expenditures on home care. Certification is another softer governing mode used to enhance competition in the Netherlands and Spain, for example (certified organizations have a higher chance of gaining a contract). Furthermore, providers' performance scores are presented to the public (naming and shaming) in England and the Netherlands; good practices are presented to the public in Finland. In the Netherlands, where competition is relatively high, there is a special organization to safeguard fair competition (the Dutch Healthcare Authority). This organization ensures the positive effects of competition through the prevention of monopolies or abuse of market power by providers or insurers. Such an organization was mentioned for no other country.

Apart from the direct quality control achieved by setting quality criteria in contracts, the contracting process is also thought to increase quality indirectly through competition. However, contracting does not always lead to competition between home-care providers. Generally, market mechanisms are scarce in Europe due to a lack of potential providers and/or the large number of publicly owned home-care providers.[8] In this context, the expansion of the number of private providers is encouraged. In Finland, for instance, partnerships between the private and publicly owned sectors are sought to cope with the growing demand for home care.

2.2.5 Concluding remarks on governance on home care

Table 2.3 provides a characterization of home-care governance as a whole – the more bullets, the stronger the governance. The final column is based on Table 2.1. Municipal and regional governments have a relatively high influence on publicly financed home care whereas the role of central governments is rather weak. Across Europe, control of needs assessment and assignment of care is used to control public provision and access to home care. Hence, it may be concluded that many governments are often involved in rowing the boat, rather than just steering it. Of course, there are differences across countries. Three main models of governance are discussed below.

2.2.6 Three types of home-care governance

Three main types of home-care governance can be defined based on the country

---
[8] For instance, in social health care in Latvia, Norway, Poland, Slovakia and Slovenia.

Table 2.3 *Overall level of (national) governance for setting a vision, involvement in regulation and integration of home-care policy*

Country	Vision[a]	Regulation	Integration of home-care policy
	●●● explicitly formulated for home care ●● for only one type of home care ● no formal document available	●●●●● national ●●●● mixed national/regional ●●● regional or mixed national/municipal ●●● mixed regional/municipal ● municipal	●●●● one ministry, one policy scheme ●●● one ministry, more schemes ●● two ministries, two schemes ● two ministries, more schemes
Austria	●●●	●●●	●●
Belgium	●●●	●●●●	●
Bulgaria	●		●
Croatia	●●●		
Cyprus	●●●	●●●●	●
Czech Republic	●●	●●●	●
Denmark	●●●	●	●●●
England	●●●	●●●	●●●
Estonia		●●●	●●
Finland	●●●	●	●●●●
France	●●●	●●●●●	●●
Germany	●●●	●●●	●●
Greece	●●●	●	
Hungary	●	●●●●	●
Iceland	●	●	●
Ireland	●●●	●●●	●●●
Italy	●●●	●	●
Latvia	●●●	●●●	●
Lithuania			●
Luxembourg	●●	●●●●●	●●
Malta	●●●	●●●●●	●●●
Netherlands	●●●	●●●	●●●
Norway	●●●	●	●●●●
Poland	●	●●	●
Portugal	●●●	●●●●●	●●
Romania	●	●●	●
Slovakia	●●●	●●●	●
Slovenia	●●	●●●	●
Spain	●●●	●●	●●
Sweden	●●●	●	●●●●
Switzerland	●●●	●●●	

[a] In the highest score, a national vision is explicitly laid down in a policy document or another formal document at national level for the whole home-care sector.

descriptions: (i) framework; (ii) centralized; and (iii) laissez-faire (see Table 2.4). The first governance type is the most common, the other two are less balanced and occur less frequently.

Framework type

This is characterized by a high level of decentralized decision-making and, at the same time, an explicit national vision on home care. Additionally, national framework regulation is applied in generally described criteria. For instance, 'people with insufficient means' or 'dependent people' are entitled to 'home care'. Furthermore, limits may be set such as setting maximum prices for home help (as in Hungary) or defining groups who need to receive at least home care free of charge. Finally, general principles are described – for example, 'the importance of quality' is stated without defining the concept 'quality'.

Municipalities and NGOs (e.g. insurance companies) can formulate more specific criteria within these general boundaries and are responsible for the organization of the system. Two examples fitting this model are found in the Netherlands and Slovenia. In the Netherlands, the national government lays down a framework regulation within which municipalities and independent agencies develop their own rules. The independent agencies 'govern' home nursing and personal-care services; municipalities regulate domestic aid. The Dutch Social Support Act provides a general description of municipal responsibilities and requires municipalities to write down a vision on social support, including domestic aid, every four years. Municipalities decide on eligibility, prices of services and the exact services that will be publicly funded. The Dutch Healthcare Authority sets maximum prices for personal care and home nursing; the Care Assessment Centre (*Centrum Indicatiestelling Zorg*) decides on the exact eligibility criteria within the boundaries of the governmental guidelines. In Slovenia, social home care is officially the municipalities' responsibility. General eligibility criteria for the publicly financed social home-care services are set in the national Rules on Standards and Norms for Social Welfare Services. These criteria are rather general so municipalities (the financing bodies) can decide to provide some services which are not provided in other regions. Social welfare institutions follow the national General Administrative Procedure Act to decide upon the rights, obligations and legal interests of individual people. Hence, this type of governance may show large intra-country differences regarding home care.

Centralized type

This is characterized by the dominant role of central government, laying down strict eligibility criteria. Regional authorities only execute the policies of the central government. This model is most pronounced in several smaller countries, but also in France and Portugal.

Laissez-faire type

Unlike the framework and the centralized types, the laissez-faire is characterized by a weak role for the central government. Typically, there is no national government vision on home care, entitlements are rarely defined and private providers and NGOs play a large role in deciding who is entitled to home care. If the government has any role it is mainly concerned with the poorest citizens and setting up a safety net. Bulgaria provides an example of this third model. A lack of governmental interference and a poor society that is unable to pay for services has led to a general lack of home care in this country. In many countries this model governs the non-public(ly financed) sector (e.g in Finland and Ireland). In Ireland, there is said to be a lack of regulation over this private sector (even that part paid through public sources) and quality assurance appears not to have been addressed so far. This facilitates more flexibility with regard to qualifications, training and monitoring of the quality of work. As a consequence, care workers in the private sector have fewer social rights than their colleagues in the public and non-profit-making sectors.

Table 2.4 *Three main types of home-care governance*

Centralized	Framework	Laissez-faire
Features		
Dominant role of national government	Non-state actors have wide decision-making power	Weak role of central government
Detailed entitlements set by national government	National vision on home care	No government vision
National vision on home care		Few entitlements
Actors		
Central government lays down detailed regulation	Central government lays down regulation along broad lines	NGOs setting their own rules or contracted sporadically by government
Municipal or regional government has main involvement in operational activities	Municipal or regional governments have large discretionary powers	Private providers setting their own rules and helping those who can afford
Private providers may be strictly regulated	NGOs may have large roles	Government for most severe cases
Main policy issues		
Efficiency	Equity	Equity
Maintaining equity		Quality in general
Examples		
Cyprus, France, Malta, Portugal	Denmark, England, Finland, Germany, Netherlands, Norway, Sweden, Switzerland	Bulgaria, Romania

The three types of governance should be understood as 'ideal types' that facilitate the understanding of the inter-country differences. Exact borders between these types cannot be drawn in practice. Besides, the situation of home-care governance in different countries is not static and they may move from one type to another. The EURHOMAP study has been cross-sectional and therefore the available data do not allow identification of developments.

2.3 Governance on home-care funding

This section addresses financing of formal home care. These services may be publicly or privately financed. When home care services are subject to public funding, this does not imply that all services are covered or that a specific service is covered fully by public resources: additional resources, such as co-payments often apply. Means testing may imply that only people below a certain level of wealth receive public funding, whereas those with a higher level of wealth pay for services completely or partially out-of-pocket. This section also pays attention to the pricing of services and the ways in which providers are funded.

In general, it is hard to determine the share of public involvement in funding home care. Data on privately financed services are missing or not comparable across countries. Still, governments' role in funding home care can be compared to some extent by comparing the funded services and co-payment requirements.

2.3.1 Services subject to public funding

The services that may be subject to public funding can be divided into several categories, such as domestic care (household chores); provision of activities of daily living (ADL) care and home nursing care; and provision of technical aids. Furthermore, there is support for undertaking activities outside the home and support for informal caregivers. No data were available for Portugal and Croatia. Social home care consists of housekeeping, shopping, transfers, household administration, transport, meals-on-wheels and social activities. Table 2.5 presents the services possibly being funded per country. However, it should be noted that the services being funded differ markedly between municipalities in many countries. Hence, this overview table does not provide the practice in each municipality but rather services that (in theory) are subject to public funding.

Domestic care

Housekeeping is partly funded in 25 countries; shopping in 22 countries. Meals-on-wheels are funded in 20 countries; help with household administration in 17 countries. However, in many countries, funding of domestic care is restricted based on the level of wealth of the recipient or his/her family. In addition, funding of this service is not always available in every municipality. For example, only some of the municipalities in Bulgaria and Finland fund domestic care. In many other countries, eligibility criteria for these services are rather strict. In the Netherlands and Poland domestic care is funded only if no family support is available. In the latter, funding of domestic care is available only to the lowest income groups. Restrictions on funding aid with household administration are mostly based on the recipient's income (as in Bulgaria, Cyprus and Poland). Sometimes municipal or regional differences exist (e.g. between Swiss cantons and between Bulgarian and Finnish municipalities). In Finland, help with household administration is a statutory right for people with severe disabilities, in contrast to domestic aid, for example. Overall, it seems that these services are covered by public funding but are often restricted to certain types of people and areas.

ADL care

Funding for assistance with washing (25 countries), dressing (26), putting on aids (25), transfers (26) and eating (25) is provided in the vast majority of the countries. However, geographical differences may exist and some countries may restrict funding to the low income group.

Nursing care

Funding of services such as changing stomas, urinal bags and help with bladder catheterization (in 26 countries); help with skin care, disinfection and prevention of bedsores (26 countries) and help with using medicines (25 countries) is also available in the majority of the countries. In Austria, funding of this type of care is limited to four weeks. In countries where municipalities are responsible for this type of care, the funding may vary by municipality (e.g. in Bulgaria and Finland). In Cyprus, funding depends on the home region and income of the recipient.

Provision of aids

The provision of a walking frame/rollator is funded in 24 countries; simple aids such as canes and crutches are publicly funded in 25 countries. Other aids (e.g. adjustable beds, wheelchairs, anti-bedsore cushions and patient lifters) are eligible for funding in 22 countries. The public contribution to the financing of aids may be income-dependent (as in Cyprus and Ireland). In Finland, aids can be rented; a loan for buying aids can be obtained in Greece; Poland offers a partial refund; and some simple aids are publicly funded in Spain (e.g. wheelchairs and walking aids).

Activities outside the home

Transportation is funded in 21 countries. Again, eligibility may vary in countries with municipal responsibilities for this type of care (e.g. Bulgaria, Finland and Latvia). Funding is income-dependent in Cyprus; means tested in

Iceland and Ireland; and co-payments are required in Spain (although there are differences in practice among the autonomous communities). Transportation is partly funded in Greece and transportation to health-care institutions is free of charge for clients with severe disabilities in Poland. Some funding is available in Switzerland but the services, controlled by special organizations, are not easily accessible. Assistance with social activities is funded in 19 countries; day-care centres provide these activities in Iceland.

Care for informal caregivers

These types of activities are the least funded in the European countries. Respite care is funded in 18 countries and counselling of relatives in 17 countries.

2.3.2 Ways of funding home care

Different types of home care (domestic aid, home nursing care, ADL assistance) may be funded differently within countries. The level of government involved in public funding can be national, regional or municipal, or a combination of these. This may also vary by type of home care.

Typically, home-care funding consists of a mixture of sources; there is seldom only one source of funding (only in Denmark, where taxation is reported as the sole source of funding). The most common sources are described below.

- Out-of-pocket payments: recipients of home care are required to pay a co-payment for care funded through taxation or social insurance. Sometimes publicly financed home care is not available or is available only to specific groups of people (e.g. very low income group). In such cases, those in need of home care who are not eligible for publicly funded care have to pay out-of-pocket.

- Taxation: may be collected at national, regional or municipal level. One general characteristic of taxation is that the collected money is not earmarked.

- Insurance: can take different forms. Home care may be funded as part of health insurance; this is mostly the case for home health care. Home care may also be funded as part of long-term care insurance or social security. All these forms of insurances can be either compulsory or voluntary. Compulsory insurance premiums are collected mostly via employees and/or employers.

- Donations and other third-party contributions: home care may be provided by charities or NGOs funded by private donations or membership fees; some countries receive funding from the EU.

Table 2.5 *Number of home-care services receiving public funding*

Country	Domestic care (max. 4 ●●●● services)	ADL care (max. 5 ●●●●● services)	Nursing care (max. 3 ●●● services)	Provision of aids (max. 4 ●●●● services)	Support for informal caregivers (max. 2 ●● services)
Austria	●●●●	●●●●●	●●	●●●●	●
Belgium[a]	●●●	●●●●●	●●●	●●●●	●●
Bulgaria[b]	●	●●●●●	●●	●●●	N/A
Croatia[c]	N/A	N/A	N/A	N/A	N/A
Cyprus[d]	●●●	●●●●	●●●	●●●●	●●
Czech Republic	●●●●	●●●●●	●●●	●●●●	●●
Denmark	●●	●●●●●	●●●	●●●●	●●
England		●●●	●●●	●●●●	●●
Estonia	●●●●	●●●●●	●●●	●●●●	●●
Finland	●●●●	●●●●●	●●●	●●●●	
France	●●●●	●●●●●	●●●	●●●●	●
Germany	●●●●	●●●●●	●●●	●●●●	●●
Greece	●●●●	●●●●●	●●●	●●●	●
Hungary[e]	N/A	N/A	●	N/A	N/A
Iceland	●●●	●●●●●	●●●	●●●●	●●
Ireland	●●●	●●●●●	●●●	●●●●	●
Italy	●●●●	●●●●●	●●●	●●●●	●
Latvia	●●●●	●●●●●	●●●	●●●●	●
Lithuania	●●●	●●●	●	●●●	N/A
Luxembourg	●●●●	●●●●	●●●	●●●●	●●
Malta	●●●●	●●●●	●●●	●●●●	●
Netherlands	●●●●	●●●●	●●●	●●●●	●●
Norway	●●●	●●●●●	●●●	●●●●	●
Poland	●●	●●●●●	●●●	●●●●	N/A
Portugal	N/A	N/A	N/A	N/A	N/A

Table 2.5 contd

Country	Domestic care (max. 4 ●●●● services)	ADL care (max. 5 ●●●●● services)	Nursing care (max. 3 ●●● services)	Provision of aids (max. 4 ●●●● services)	Support for informal caregivers (max. 2 ●● services)
Romania	●●	●●●	●	N/A	N/A
Slovakia	●●●●	●●●●●	●●	●●●●	●●
Slovenia	●●●	●●●●●	●●●	●●	●
Spain	●●●	●●●●●	●●●	●●●●	●●
Sweden	●●	●●●●●	●●●	●●●●	●
Switzerland	●●●●	●●●●●	●●●	●●●	●
Includes:	housekeeping, shopping, administration, meals-on-wheels	washing, dressing, eating, putting on aids, transfers	stoma, skin care, medicine	provision of rollator, adaptation of dwelling, simple aids, other aids	respite care, counselling of relatives

[a] Data for Flanders only; [b] These services are publicly funded in very few municipalities; [c] No data available for social home care; [d] Nursing care is publicly funded in only a few areas; [e] Home help, social catering (meals-on-wheels), physiotherapy, shipment of medical devices, telecare and home adaptations are publicly funded in some regions; N/A: no information available.

Taxation is one of the sources of funding in all countries except Germany (Table 2.6 highlights the most important sources of funding). For almost all of the countries that use taxation as a source of funding, state level taxation is used to fund home care to at least some extent (27 countries – Table 2.6 sets the most important level at which funding was collected in bold).[9] In Europe, generally the municipalities provide (extra) funding for home care through taxation. The regional level is involved in several countries (e.g. Belgium, Croatia, Sweden and Switzerland).

Social (health) insurance can often be found in place beside taxation. In that case, home health care is financed mostly via the (health) insurance system and social health care via taxation. This is the case in the Netherlands, Poland, Slovenia, Slovakia, Switzerland and partially in Belgium. The situation is reversed in Portugal and Sweden – home health care is funded via taxation and social health care via social security and taxation. In Luxembourg, both types of home care are funded by a combination of obligatory insurance and a state contribution based on taxes. There are 23 countries where (obligatory) insurance was mentioned as a source of funding. This may be a health insurance or a social security insurance (see Table 2.6). Belgium (Flanders only), Germany, Luxembourg and the Netherlands have specific compulsory care insurances for long-term care, including home care.

There are a few peculiarities in the sources of home-care funding: *EU-funding* is mentioned in Bulgaria and Greece (see Table 2.6, third-party contributions). Until recently, EU funding covered up to 75% of the costs in Greece. *Donations* are mentioned in Bulgaria, Cyprus, Greece, Lithuania, Portugal, Romania and Slovenia.

Home-care funding may stem from the social security budget or the health-care budget. Where home care is (partly) funded under the health-care budget, percentages range widely in Europe. Seven countries[10] in our study allocated over 5% of the total health-care expenditure to home care. Most countries (11)[11] spend between 1% and 5% of their health budget. For eight countries[12] no information is available on expenditure on home care as a proportion of total health-care expenditure. Six of these countries[13] have data on part of their home-care spending but these cannot be related to total health-care expenditure. As home care is not always part of the health-care system, large differences are found between social home care and home health care as a percentage of GDP. For total home care this ranges from 0.02% in Latvia to 0.70% in the

---
9 In Denmark, Latvia and Switzerland taxation for home care is levied at regional or municipal level, not at national level.
10 Austria, Belgium, Denmark, Germany, Luxembourg, Norway and Poland.
11 Czech Republic, England, Finland, France, Lithuania, Malta, the Netherlands, Portugal, Romania, Spain and Sweden.
12 Croatia, Greece, Iceland, Ireland, Italy, Latvia, Slovenia and Switzerland.
13 Iceland, Ireland, Italy, Latvia, Slovenia and Switzerland.

Fig. 2.1 *Home-care expenditures*[a] *as a proportion of GDP*

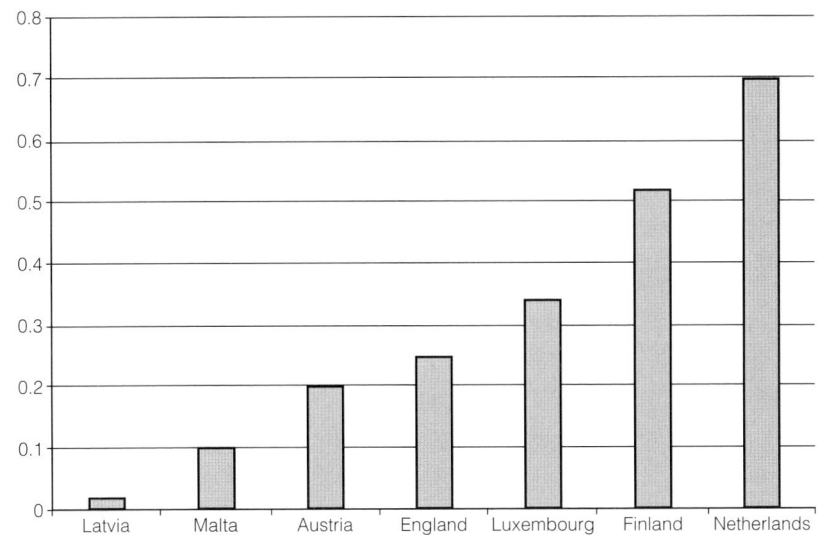

[a] Including long-term care, help with IADL and rehabilitative and curative care at home.

Note: comparable data containing all the expenditure elements were available for only these seven countries and for different years (as shown).

Source: country reports (www.nivel.eu/eurhomap).

Netherlands (see Fig. 2.1). Some countries spend most on home health care; others spend more on home help. One explanation is the differences in the financing of personal care which can be part of social home care or of home health care. In general, Denmark, the Netherlands, Norway and Sweden – but also Greece, Poland and Romania – spend relatively (as a share of GDP) the most on home care.

Data on *private expenditure* for home health care (long-term, rehabilitative and curative care) as a share of total health-care expenditure are available for 20 countries.[14] With the exception of Cyprus, private expenditures are less than public expenditures on home health care in all these countries. However, considerable data are missing. For instance, the nursing service in Cyprus has been widely developed over recent years but is not taken up in the international databases. Furthermore, private expenditures seem to be incomplete or missing in many countries. The data that could be retrieved showed that (apart from Cyprus) the countries with the highest shares of private expenditure are Belgium (21%) and Spain (24%). There seems to be a strong polarization: between 5% and 15% of home care is privately financed in only four countries; eleven countries show private expenditure below 5% of total home-care expenditure. It is important to note that the Eurostat and OECD data refer only to the

---

14 Austria, Belgium, Bulgaria, Croatia, Czech Republic, Denmark, Estonia, Finland, Germany, Hungary, Iceland, Lithuania, Luxembourg, Norway, Poland, Spain, Slovakia, Slovenia, Romania and Sweden.

Table 2.6 Funding of formal home care[a]

Country	Public funding mechanism				Private funding mechanism		
	Taxation Level: national, regional, municipal		Insurance[b] Type: social, health, care		Third-party contributions[c] • = yes	Co-payments/ private payments[d] Means tested: yes, partly, no	
	Social home care	Home health care	Social home care	Home health care		Social home care	Home health care
Austria	n, r, m			h		• n	• n
Belgium	r, m		c	h	•	• y	• y
Bulgaria	**n**, m	m, **n**		h	•	• y	• y (part)
Croatia	n	n, r		h		• y	• n (part)
Cyprus	n	n		s	•	• y (part)	• y (part)
Czech Republic	**n**, r, m			h		• y (part)	
Denmark	n, **m**	n, **m**					• n (part)
England	**n**, m	**n**, m				• y	• y (part)
Estonia	**m**	n		h			• y (part)
Finland	n, m	n, m	s	s		• y	• y
France	n, **r**	n	h	h		• y	• n
Germany			c	h		• n	
Greece	n	n		s	•	• y	•
Hungary	m			h		• y	•
Iceland	n	n				• y	• y
Ireland	n	n				• y	• y
Italy	**n**, r, m	**n**, r, m				• y	• y
Latvia	m			h[e]		• y	• n
Lithuania	n, **m**	n		h	•		• n
Luxembourg	n, m	n	c	h		• y (part)	• n
Malta	n	n				• n	• n
Netherlands	**n**, m	n	c	c		• y	• y
Norway	n, m	n, m				• y	
Poland	n, **r**, **m**	n	s	h		• y	
Portugal		n	s		•	• y	
Romania	n, **m**		h	h	•	• y	•
Slovakia	n, **m**	n		h		• y	
Slovenia	m	m		h	•	• y	
Spain	**n, r,** m	n				• y	
Sweden	m	m, r	s			• (part)	
Switzerland	**r**, m	n		h		• y	• n

[a] Predominant mode of funding is printed in bold; [b] care insurance comprises specific long-term care insurance or home-care insurance; [c] donations and a few cases of EU contributions; [d] indicates presence of private or co-payments; [e] mixed tax–insurance system.

expenditure on home care that is considered to be part of the health-care expenditure – in most cases this covers only home nursing care and ADL care. Indications could be retrieved for home help in some countries – the highest share in Slovenia (40%); Austria and Germany both showed 27%; Luxembourg was just 1.3%. There are large differences between home nursing and home help (e.g. in the Czech Republic, Finland and Slovenia), with relatively more private payments for home help. However, most only referred to co-payments rather than completely privately funded care (for an example, compare data for Finland in Eurostat and data found through this study for all private payments).

There seems to be no relation between the number of services subject to public funding and the type of funding in a country. Both the level of taxation (national, regional or municipal) and the type of insurance (health, social or no insurance) appear to have no relation to the number of services that are publicly funded.

2.3.3 Methods for paying providers

There are several ways of funding home-care providers. They may receive a (fixed) budget or be remunerated by salaries or fee-for-service. Often, there is a differentiation in the 'intensity of care'. Mills and Ranson (2006) discuss the advantages and disadvantages of different payment methods in the healthcare sector. Funding through salaries has the disadvantage that providers may restrict the number of patients and services provided. Also, it will probably be a disincentive in low-income countries as the level of payment is usually low. The solution is to include performance-related pay or non-financial incentives (such as certificates). Under fixed budgets, providers are paid for all services provided by a facility in a given time period but they may reduce the number of patients and services provided and keep patients longer. A monitoring system would address such actions and the possible lack of quality (Mills & Ranson, 2006). This system has the advantage of enabling better control of costs and stimulating preventive and psychosocial care (Hutten & Kerkstra, 1996). Fee-for-service is paid for each act or visit and may, for instance, relate to hours of care provided or the number of clients who received care. The disadvantage is that it may lead to overprovision of (more expensive) services; the advantage is that patients may have greater freedom of choice. Under capitation/block contracts, providers are paid for all relevant services for a patient in a given time period. This has the advantage of stimulating continuity of care and encouraging preventive services. However, providers may reduce contacts per patient and service intensity. Finally, case payments (payments per type of patient) may be used, with the disadvantage that providers may decrease service intensity and provide less expensive services.

Two types of payment method for funding-providing agencies can be distinguished. Publicly funded home health care agencies are generally paid either by fee-for-service (14 countries)[15] or through fixed budgets (11

---

[15] Belgium, Czech Republic, Denmark, England, Estonia, Hungary, Latvia, Luxembourg, Netherlands, Norway, Portugal, Romania, Slovakia and Slovenia.

countries)[16] and sometimes a combination of both (Belgium). *Fee-for-service* may be paid per unit of time (Luxembourg, Norway, Romania, Slovenia, Switzerland and for home health care in Poland), per visit (Latvia), per service delivered (Iceland) or based on the number of care packages to be provided (England, the Netherlands). In Luxembourg, the fee is based on care intensity and level of competence required. The budget can be based on the number of services (Ireland, Lithuania) or the number of inhabitants or insured people (Bulgaria, Greece, Hungary, Norway, Slovakia). *Negotiated budgets* exist in Malta. Different types of payment can be found in Germany, where the market sets prices as agencies sell care to their clients. A similar situation exists in Austria, where those in receipt of care benefits have to pay the providers. In some countries (e.g. Cyprus and Switzerland) care providers are in the salaried service of the authorities. Private home health-care services (i.e. not funded under the public scheme) are most often paid fee-for-service and clients pay the providing agencies directly, with no involvement of governmental agencies.

Agencies providing social home-care services are publicly funded either through a fee-for-service system (14 countries)[17] or by fixed budgets (10 countries).[18] Fee-for-service can be based on hours (6 countries);[19] number of services provided (Hungary); or number of clients (Greece). Intensity of care is included in the fee in England, Italy and the Netherlands. Fixed budgets may be based on some kind of capitation (Bulgaria and Finland). Municipalities set the budget in several countries. Negotiated budgets between financers and providers of social care exist in England, Malta and Poland, for example. In the Netherlands, payment of providers of personal and nursing care at home is based on 'functions' (packages of services) and 'performance levels'. In at least seven countries,[20] informal caregivers can receive financial compensation.

2.3.4 Price setting and contributions for clients

The country reports were intended to provide information on both price-setting mechanisms (i.e. procedures used at national/regional level to determine the price for home-care providers' services) and on the level of contributions (i.e. fees) required from final users/clients. Unfortunately, in many cases only one of these two aspects has been clarified within the national reports. In part this reflects the lack of clarity on the political and/or technical processes underlying price setting in home care in some countries. One commonality for both price

---

16 Bulgaria, Croatia, Finland, France, Greece, Iceland, Ireland, Italy, Lithuania, Malta and Poland.
17 Belgium, Denmark, England, Greece, Hungary, Italy, Luxembourg, Netherlands, Norway, Poland, Portugal, Romania, Slovenia and Switzerland.
18 Bulgaria, Croatia, Czech Republic, Estonia, Finland, France, Iceland, Ireland, Lithuania and Malta.
19 Norway, Poland, Portugal, Romania, Slovenia and Switzerland.
20 Bulgaria, Cyprus, Finland, Luxembourg, the Netherlands, Romania and some wealthier regions of Italy.

and contribution setting for home care is that, in many countries, these depend on the characteristics of the:

- care provided: type of care, time of provision, personnel involved, materials and technical aid required; and the

- care recipient: functional and cognitive level of dependency (e.g. ADL, IADL), socioeconomic situation (personal or family income) and place of living (e.g. rural/urban, wealthy/poor region).

Prices are not often set at the national level. In several countries providers are contracted by (health) care insurance companies or municipalities and, in some cases, they set the prices. Each contractor uses different prices. Prices are set (for example) for home nursing in Estonia, Hungary and Slovenia and for most home-care services in Iceland. Little information is available on the basis of calculation but some price-setting processes were identified. In France, prices are set through both a technical evaluation (e.g. in terms of a standard time and the tariffs for personnel) and a negotiation between providers and the funding institution at national level. Luxembourg uses a similar process, involving the umbrella organization of care providers. In the Netherlands, the Dutch Healthcare Authority sets maximum prices by considering labour costs, level of expertise required, productivity and overheads – these prices are index-linked. In Germany, prices are negotiated between representatives of care providers and long-term care institutions. The Lithuanian report states that "the Ministry of Health sets the prices for home health care after the evaluation of the Board of the State Patient Fund and the Compulsory Health Insurance." This suggests that the negotiation of prices includes both political and technical issues.

In some countries, the municipal level has a high degree of autonomy in negotiating the price of social home care directly with providers – as in the Scandinavian countries (e.g. Denmark, Finland and Sweden), Slovakia and Switzerland. But even where there is freedom to decide the prices of (some) home-care services, some central governments have set national guidelines for price setting (e.g. social home care in Slovenia). In Spain, prices vary among the autonomous communities and the lack of recognition of home-care prices is now considered to be a demanding governance problem.

In most countries (24) clients must contribute out-of-pocket for publicly provided home care. This may be either because they are not eligible for free care – for instance due to income limits, as in Greece, Italy, Latvia, Slovenia and for social home care in Poland – or because all clients are required to make a co-payment, which can be means tested. Such means testing of client co-payments is common (19 of the 24 countries), based mostly on the income of the recipient or his/her family. Sometimes the number of people in a household is part of the means testing. In Portugal, for example, the co-payment for social home care is 50–60% of the income per capita of the household.

Free-of-charge services are provided in Bulgaria and, for social home care, in Poland but only for those on very low incomes. In Denmark and Sweden most services are also free of charge and long-term home care is a universal right that is not means tested. Health services are more often free of charge than social-care services. Free home-health services are provided in, for instance, Ireland, Norway, Poland, Slovenia and Spain. The opposite is true for Luxembourg where domestic care and personal care are free of charge and home health care is subject to co-payments.

2.3.5 Possible types of home-care financing

Home-care funding is characterized mainly by the wide variation in how financing is organized. However, there seem to be two main *types of home-care funding*. The first is a combination of taxation for social home care and health insurance for home nursing care. The second is a combination of taxation for home nursing care and social insurance for social home care. Within these models, there are wide variations in how funding mechanisms are organized in practice. Only three countries have a specific care insurance in place.

The *contribution of clients* can be divided into three different types. First, the free-of-charge type in which home care is financed fully from public money, leaving no co-payments for individual clients (as in Denmark). Secondly, the means tested co-payments type. This can be divided into means testing with the aim either to contribute more when income is higher or to provide care free of charge for those with low incomes, resulting in fully out-of-pocket payments for those above the income ceiling. Thirdly, the fixed co-payment type, which requires clients to pay a fixed amount or percentage of the fee. These models usually differ between home health care and social home care within countries.

Little is known about the privately financed home-care sector although this is the main provider of home care in many countries, especially in eastern Europe, Portugal and Greece. Expenditures on social home care are often part of the social security budget. Data on the expenditure seem rarely collected and total expenditure on home care is seldom available. Hardly any data are available for care financed under social security and private care.

2.4 Challenges and developments

In Europe, governments have large control over the home-care sector although there are some exceptions, such as Bulgaria and Romania. Many governments are involved in rowing the boat (i.e. providing care and assessing individual care needs) instead of steering the boat (i.e. providing the conditions for other organizations to provide home care). However, financial constraints may drive the role more towards steering private organizations (i.e. through setting requirements for the quality of care and access to care). Several country experts interviewed for this study mentioned the lack of regulation on the private sector as one of their main concerns. Hence, future governments will likely be concerned with regulating privately owned home-care providers and less involved in actual provision and needs assessment.

Concerns were expressed about the lack of national-level regulation of the home-care sector and about inadequate regulations. The lack of national policies has led to equity problems in Finland, Latvia and Romania. Furthermore, there was said to be a lack of control over the quality of care in several countries.[21] The concerns about inadequate regulations included overlapping regulations (as in Belgium); too-detailed regulations (e.g. organizational requirements for receipt of public funding in Portugal); excessive paperwork (e.g. in Denmark, Finland and the Netherlands); and unfair regulations (i.e. different financing rules for different types of home-care provider as in Belgium, Latvia and Slovakia).

Other frequently mentioned problems are separate policies and financing mechanisms for home nursing and home help. These are possibly affecting the accessibility of services and the quality and efficiency of care provision. Poor coordination of delivery was reported for Belgium, Italy, Lithuania, Poland, Spain and Sweden. In Spain, however, the situation varies by autonomous community – some communities show good practices but others have no coordination. Coordination may be undermined by, for example, unclear division of responsibilities (as in Hungary) and separate funding systems (as in Latvia and Poland).

Data on expenditures on home care are necessary for adequate steering. At present, there is insufficient information and indicators are non-comparable. Many countries[22] reported a lack of funding for home care. For instance, home care in Bulgaria and Greece depended on foreign financial capital, hence there are concerns that the drying up of these foreign financial resources may lead to the breakdown of home-care programmes. In Denmark, Finland, Hungary and Latvia some, mainly smaller and remote, municipalities have cut home-care services as a result of financial shortages. Cash benefits for home care were said to be too low to cover needs in Austria, Hungary and for adults with disabilities in Germany. Also, publicly financed home-care

---

21 In Belgium, France, Ireland, Italy, Latvia and Switzerland.
22 Bulgaria, Greece, Ireland, Italy, Luxembourg, Slovakia and Slovenia.

services were said to be too expensive in several other countries.[23] With ageing populations, governments may need to reconsider the affordability of a largely publicly funded home-care system. The unavailability of dedicated funding for home care was a further concern – that is, the home-care budget's position as a non-earmarked part of general practice or primary care could lead to underfunding of home care and problems with access to the home-care market for non-GP-related providers.

The experts mentioned developments in home care regarding changes in the policy instruments used: decentralizing decision-making powers to municipal or regional governments in some countries (social home care in Cyprus, the Czech Republic and the Netherlands, and planned in Lithuania and Romania) and centralizing these powers in others (e.g. home nursing in Cyprus and planned in Finland); and increasing transparency in expenditures. Many countries are engaged in introducing new funding mechanisms for home care (in at least 12 countries). The reasons for introducing such new mechanisms are diverse – some are meant to increase equity,[24] others are intended to stimulate coordination between home care and hospital care (as in Germany) or to secure financing of home care.[25] In Poland (disability insurance), England and in some local contexts in Italy (personal budgets) these plans pertain to cash rather than in-kind benefits, giving the clients a more central role in organizing their care. Client co-payments have been introduced in Romania and Switzerland. A basic insurance package will also be introduced in Romania. In Slovenia and Spain long-term care insurances are being introduced. Voluntary insurances are planned in several countries (i.e. Croatia and Slovenia). Thus, much is changing in the area of financing home care. In addition to these changes in financing mechanisms, greater transparency on home-care expenditures has become a policy focus in some countries.[26]

Investing in the client-centredness of home care is a common policy (in Denmark, England, Germany, the Netherlands and Slovakia). This is done through taking up client-centredness as a measured quality norm, through *outcome*-based financing (providers are paid on the basis of measurable outcomes grounded on goals set jointly by the client and professional staff) and by providing clients with quality information about providers or promoting client choice in general.

All in all, home-care governance is in full transition, including changes to financing mechanisms and political centralization or decentralization.

---

23 For example, England, Croatia, France, Hungary, Poland and Slovakia.
24 In Croatia, Italy, Latvia, Slovakia and Switzerland.
25 In Estonia, Latvia, Poland and Romania.
26 In Belgium, Croatia, Finland and the Netherlands.

References

Bettio F, Plantenga J (2004). Comparing care regimes in Europe. *Feminist Economics*, 10(1):85–113.

Billings J, Leichsenring K, eds. (2005). *Integrating health and social care services for older persons: evidence from nine European countries.* Aldershot, Ashgate Publishing Limited (Public Policy and Social Welfare Series, Vol. 31).

Burau V, Theobald H, Blank R (2007). *Governing home care: a cross national comparison.* Cheltenham, Edward Elgar Publishing.

Colombo F et al. (2011). *Help wanted? Providing and paying for long-term care.* Paris, Organisation for Economic Co-operation and Development (OECD Health Policy Studies).

Governance Working Group of the International Institute of Administrative Sciences (1996). *Defining urban governance.* Kobe, Global Development Research Center (http://www.gdrc.org/u-gov/governance-define.html, accessed 6 June 2012).

Hutten JBF, Kerkstra A (1996). *Home care in Europe: a country-specific guide to its organization and financing.* Aldershot, Ashgate.

Mills AJ, Ranson MK (2006). The design of health systems. In: Merson MH, Black RE, Mills A. *International public health: diseases, programs, systems and policies.* Sudbury, Jones & Bartlett:513–547.

Mossialos E et al. (2002). *Funding health care – options for Europe.* Buckingham, Open University Press (European Observatory on Health Care Systems Series).

RVZ (2005). *Langdurige zorg verzekerd [Long-term care insured].* The Hague, Council on Public Health and Health Care.

Saltman RB, Bankauskaite V, Vrangbaek K, eds. (2007). *Decentralization in health care: strategies and outcomes.* Maidenhead, Open University Press (European Observatory on Health Systems and Policies series).

Viitanen T (2007). *Informal and formal care in Europe.* Sheffield: University of Sheffield and IZA (Discussion paper No. 2648).

Chapter 3
Clients in focus

Vjenka Garms-Homolová, Michel Naiditch, Cecilia Fagerström, Giovanni Lamura, Maria Gabriella Melchiorre, László Gulácsi, Allen Hutchinson

3.1 Introduction

It is not always easy to obtain appropriate home care. The Special Eurobarometer study of 2007 reflected European citizens' worries about their old age and access to care in the case of dependency (TNS Opinion & Social, 2007). A large proportion of respondents expected that the care needs of their aged relatives would not be covered appropriately in the future. Still, a majority of the respondents in the Special Eurobarometer survey believed that the state should provide home-care services and pay for required care, at least to some extent (TNS Opinion & Social, 2007). About half of the respondents believed that adult children should be required to contribute financially to care for their parents (TNS Opinion & Social, 2007). Also, should they become frail in older age, the respondents would prefer to live with their children (45% of EU respondents to the Eurobarometer questionnaire). The availability and the role of informal care – in this case care provided voluntarily – is a central factor that can explain differences in the overall role of home care in Europe. When informal caregivers are not available, formal care services are important to meet home-care needs. Moreover, public attitudes towards informal care logically will influence both the willingness of family members to provide informal services and the availability of formal care services.

Across Europe, informal care is thought to be decreasing. Smaller family sizes may lead to fewer potential informal caregivers. Increasing female participation in the labour force (Genre, Salvador & Lamo, 2011) also may reduce the time available for informal care. Viitanen (2005) found that providing informal care for elderly people decreased women's participation in the labour market.

This chapter will examine the accessibility of home care and the actual recipients of these services. Furthermore, it will discuss informal care. This is often the preferred way of care among those needing help and the availability of family care is seen as a precondition for home care in many countries. The chapter focuses on clients' and their informal caregivers' access to organized, professional home care; the clients' role in the home-care structure; and the possible problems for clients within the system. This study has focused on the structure and organization of home care and thus may add to the insight on the existing variation in the views and opinions of clients and their informal carers and the related variations in the organization of home care. As in the rest of the book, in this chapter home care refers to formal, needs-assessed care.

3.2 Clients

3.2.1 Users of home care and their opinions on accessibility

The lack of standardization of health and social care data constitutes a major difficulty for comparing home-care clients across countries. There are three main reasons. First, the definitions of home care differ across countries. Secondly, data from different countries measure outcomes for differing lengths of time (some refer to one day, others to a week, and still others to a year). Thirdly, no data on home-care recipients were available in many countries. In particular, the utilization rate of home care differs widely across countries. Looking at seven countries,[1] the smallest share of people served by home care was found in Croatia and the largest shares in the Netherlands and Sweden. The utilization rate ranges from 0.3% to 4.8% of the total population. Even though these client data should be interpreted with caution, they are nevertheless a first attempt at comparing the relative "generosity" of countries in terms of home-care provision. The OECD Health Data (OECD, 2010)[2] show that the public system of long-term care at home (excluding help with IADL) is most generous in Norway and Sweden and least generous in Poland and Italy. When considering only people over the age of 65, Austria, the Netherlands and Norway cover the largest share; Poland and Italy cover the smallest.

Help with ADL and IADL in 13 European countries[3] was provided to the largest share of the population in Sweden, the Netherlands and Norway; and to the smallest share in Slovenia, Cyprus and Estonia. Data measured over a year in seven countries[4] show Slovakia, Bulgaria and Poland to have low coverage

---

1 Croatia, Denmark, England, Italy, the Netherlands, Norway and Sweden.

2 These data refer to people receiving some type of personal care or nursing services delivered in any "home-like setting" by "paid workers", whether professional or not.

3 Belgium (Flanders only), Cyprus, Denmark, Estonia, Finland, France, Greece, Ireland, Luxembourg, the Netherlands, Norway, Slovenia and Sweden.

4 Bulgaria, Latvia, Lithuania, Malta, Poland, Portugal and Slovakia.

rates, ranging from 0.1% to 2.4% of the total population (in these countries the data referred to users over an entire year; in the other countries they referred to a certain month or day). Among the seven countries with available data on the population over 65 years of age,[5] the share of population receiving long-term help with ADL or nursing at home was largest in Austria, the Netherlands and Denmark; and lowest in Luxembourg and Germany. Each of these indicators shows that home care seems more comprehensive in the Scandinavian countries and the Netherlands and least comprehensive in eastern Europe.

However, data from another study that measured the hours of home care provided, rather than the percentage of the population covered by home care, point to different conclusions.[6] Measuring the hours of professional home help per week provided to people over the age of 50 in 14 countries,[7] the median was highest in Switzerland and Austria (5 hours) and lowest in Sweden (3 hours) and Denmark (1 hour). The results were different for home nursing – the median was lowest in Sweden, France and Denmark and highest in Greece (30.5 hours) and Germany (6 hours). It is possible that the medians in the Scandinavian countries are low because people with a low level of need are eligible for home-care services. In the other countries these services are provided only to clients with a high level of need and informal caregivers usually help those with lower levels of need. These seemingly contradictory results show that eligibility for services differs across countries. In some countries, policies focus on basic care for all (Scandinavian countries); in others (Germany, Italy), policies emphasize intensive help and care for the few individuals with the highest levels of need.

The Special Eurobarometer survey showed that about one quarter of the respondents in Europe worry about access to, and the quality of, home-care services. One quarter of the surveyed population considered the quality of health care provided at home to be insufficient; about two fifths characterized it as good, and one third was unable to assess the quality (TNS Opinion & Social, 2007). Similar results were obtained for health care provided in nursing homes. One quarter of the respondents expected that it would be difficult to access services, whereas about two fifths thought it was going to be easy. Affordability and the selection of health care will be discussed in section 3.3.

In almost all countries, more people receive (and prefer) long-term home care than institutional care. The exception is Slovenia, where institutional care is preferred for dependent elderly people (TNS Opinion & Social, 2007). The reason for these differing preferences is unknown; further research may be able to clarify the special situation in Slovenia.

---

5 Denmark, Finland, Germany, Luxembourg, the Netherlands, Norway and Sweden.
6 SHARE (2009) (version 3.0.1; own calculation).
7 Austria, Belgium, Czech Republic, Denmark, Finland, France, Germany, Greece, Ireland, Italy, the Netherlands, Spain, Sweden and Switzerland.

3.2.2 Voice and responsibilities of users of home-care services

It is not known to what extent clients can influence the provision and quality of care. The EURHOMAP data cannot fully answer this question. Nevertheless, some indications can be provided, especially in countries where clients receive cash benefits, rather than benefits in service. Today, benefits in service or personal budgets are available in many countries (e.g. Belgium, Cyprus, the Czech Republic, Denmark, England, Finland, France and the Netherlands). In these countries, people are able to choose the providers and even the type of care, unless there is a shortage or even absence of providers. In such cases the only option is to hire non-professionals. In some countries, receipt of cash benefits places a lot of responsibility on clients and their relatives. For example, in Austria and the Czech Republic clients are responsible for finding and buying their own services. The German system is different – benefits in cash, which are lower than benefits in kind, are available only for reimbursing care by relatives.

Clients also have the opportunity to influence the quality of care. In many countries, service providers are obliged to give clients the chance to complain. This topic is covered in the next chapter (Section 4.6).

3.3 Access to home care

This section summarizes factors promoting or hindering access to home-care services in 31 European countries.

3.3.1 Conceptualization and measures of access and accessibility

In the existing literature, there is no precise definition of the terms 'access' and 'accessibility'. Gulliford, Figueroa-Munoz and Morgan (2003) remind us that, traditionally, access to health care has been conceptualized and measured in terms of physical availability. In the mid 1970s, researchers and policy-makers started to pay attention to personal, organizational and financial barriers that can arise when certain groups of individuals want to utilize services (Millmann, 1993). At the same time, the fit between the patient and the system and the processes of the production and utilization of care became important (Penchansky & Thomas, 1981). Researchers turned to difficulties in reaching services; collective or individual ability to travel; incentives; and decision-making on the meso-level. Since the 1980s, psychological aspects have also been considered, such as consumers' perception, information status, help-seeking behaviour, ability to recognize their own needs, and expectations. While 'access' is used mainly for 'external factors' (e.g. proximity, regulations), 'accessibility' often refers to factors concerned with individual abilities and preconditions to obtaining access, such as affordability, information, choice and decision-making. However, no clear distinction seems to be possible.

Several aspects of access are the subjects of other chapters in this book (for example, in those on governance, financing and quality). This section focuses on the following topics – eligibility and entitlement; allocation versus free choice; affordability of home-care services; and geographical determinants of access to home care. Additionally, some psychological factors, such as individual experiences and the motivation of potential clients and their relatives to obtain and accept care, will be discussed (Section 3.4).

3.3.2 Eligibility and entitlement [8]

In all 31 countries, some kind of reimbursement or benefit already exists or is on the way, even though this development has not yet progressed very far in countries such as Bulgaria and Romania. However, in many countries with a fully developed system, entitlement rarely results in the opening of doors to comprehensive home care. One reason is the division of home care into two parts – health care and social care. This division is in place in most countries in Europe. Usually, each part of care is covered by different financial sources (see Chapter 2) and therefore different rules govern eligibility, allocation and administration. In some countries, the eligibility criteria for both social and health care are similar (Norway); in others, they are not fully congruent; and in other countries still, sophisticated criteria of eligibility and claim entitlement exist for one type of service only. This is the case in Austria and Italy, for example. Citizens of Sweden and Denmark, where home care is "a universal right", seem to face fewer problems than most with regards to eligibility. In a few countries, no uniform criteria of eligibility have been developed so far. For example, access to services seems to be determined arbitrarily in Bulgaria and Greece.

Difficulties of access are reported from countries in which people with physical, mental and affective impairments are not treated equally. Sometimes, a certain type of need is neglected. For instance, in Poland, only individuals severely impaired in ADL are eligible for home care; in Germany and Estonia, physical impairment is also much more important for the eligibility assessment than depression or cognitive impairment. People who are 'only' depressed or cognitively impaired receive a lower degree of benefits than those impaired in ADL. Belgium has created a special budget for people with dementia and a similar development is on the way in other countries (e.g. Germany).

---

8 Eligibility for home care from the policy-maker's perspective is described in Chapter 2.

3.3.3 Allocation, choice and information

Currently, most European countries have in place allowance systems for home care under which people with diseases and impairments are eligible for benefits in kind. In some countries, only cash benefits (also called direct payment or personal-care budget) are available – as in Austria and the Czech Republic. Recipients can then access home care as paying customers and assemble an individual package of services based on their specific needs. Both types of benefits are provided in some European states. For example, in France, Germany and the Netherlands potential users have a choice between both options.

Each type of benefit has both advantages and disadvantages. In theory, direct payment guarantees client choice and adaptation to the individual situation. In reality, many users may not be in a position either to recognize their needs properly or to find the services that they require. Choice works best if appropriate information is available and if clients are able to use the information and understand how the system works. Some information gaps were reported from the majority of the countries that participated in this study but there are examples of good practice. In the Netherlands, many initiatives have been undertaken to increase clients' knowledge on the availability of home-care services. For instance, special 'centres' in municipalities and a national-level web site were set up to inform people where and how they can apply for care. The co-payment process also seems to lack transparency. A solution to the lack of information available to users has been found in Iceland, where some counselling is offered to make the assessment process more transparent. However, people with lower educational levels and various social problems are disadvantaged in access to information.

Some country reports indicated that clients are unable to take the role of employer of their caregivers. However, this role is required only when people use a direct payment. Benefits in kind have the disadvantage of low flexibility and the fact that, for a variety of reasons, often they do not correspond with clients' individual needs, as reported in England, France and Germany. Also, the allocation policy for home nursing (health services) and for home care (social services) frequently differs since home nursing is usually only accessible for specific conditions or illness, and sometimes the timespan of provision is limited (e.g. after hospital discharge, as in Austria and Germany).

Professional case management is used in some countries to support access and utilization of home care (as in Ireland) but this kind of support is available rather rarely. Case management can also restrict freedom of choice. In England, case management is in place in many regions but the choice may not be that of the client but rather that of the case manager who decides on eligibility.

Generally, many countries are intensifying their efforts to inform citizens about the availability of services and how to obtain them. Some prefer a unique point of entry or try to deliver specific and tailored information as well as counselling to clients and their families. Examples can be found in France, the Netherlands and the Scandinavian countries (see also Chapter 4). Still, the information provided does not include all aspects necessary to improve the decision-making abilities of families seeking services.

3.3.4 Affordability of services

Although some reimbursement for the provision of services or some cash benefits exist in most of the countries, a number of economic factors restrict affordability and consequently access to home care in many parts of Europe. In only a few countries (e.g. Denmark, Luxembourg and Sweden) can a great part of individual needs be covered with publicly funded professional care. Mainly, benefits are intended to cover only essential needs, as in Hungary and Germany. Everything that exceeds the 'basics' (a certain amount of hours of care) has to be covered by the clients. Additionally, a co-payment is necessary – in some countries for all services, in others for only a part (e.g Italy). If a special need has to be covered, a large co-payment may be needed, depending on financial eligibility (as in England). The requirement to pay represents a barrier to utilization for some groups of people in many states. A further obstacle is the increasing price of services or of the wages of staff. While clients' expenditures are growing continuously, the cash benefits remain the same. Thus, their purchasing power is decreasing (as in France and Germany) and a larger co-payment becomes necessary (as in Italy).

In the framework of the Special Eurobarometer survey, European citizens were asked their opinion on the affordability of services for themselves or for their relatives. About 30% considered home health care to be affordable but another 30% thought that it would be too expensive. Expectations varied widely between countries (TNS Opinion & Social, 2007). There were very high proportions of respondents who believed that home care was not affordable in Portugal, Croatia and Greece (ranging from 56% to 71%). The largest shares of respondents who thought that home care was affordable or that it was free of charge were found in Belgium, Denmark, France and the Netherlands (42% to 59% respectively).

3.3.5 Geographically bounded determinants of access and infrastructure disparities

Geographical factors influence access in multiple ways. First, there are huge differences in the density of home-care networks across Europe. There seems to be not only a north to south gradient but also a west to east gradient. This means that countries such as Denmark, England, France, Germany, the Netherlands, Norway, Sweden and the Flanders region in Belgium offer a dense network of home care. Countries on the south-eastern rim of Europe (e.g. Bulgaria, Cyprus, Romania and Slovakia) have the thinnest care networks in the EU and care of ill or frail people is the responsibility of informal carers. Secondly, the availability of services differs within countries too. Mountains, sea, sparse road and transportation networks also represent barriers for the delivery of care to those with homes in remote places. In such regions, home visits by physicians and mobile rehabilitation services are restricted, as in the Czech Republic.

In countries with a federal or decentralized administration (e.g. in Austria and Belgium) there are considerable differences between different regional or municipal authorities. For instance, in Belgium the rules of the federal government apply to the whole country but their implementation may vary from one administrative unit to another. Accessibility is good in some parts but less good in others. A considerable gap between urban and rural areas was observed in the majority of countries (e.g. in Bulgaria, Latvia and Lithuania and for certain medical programmes in the Czech Republic). Rural areas show a lack of services, poor infrastructure and limited availability of professional caregivers. One reason may be migration towards cities or western Europe (as in the Czech Republic), but also the fact that more staff are needed to bridge the distances (as in Bulgaria).

Often, the inhabitants of villages and small communities do not have sufficient opportunity to use either home care or home nursing or other health and social services (as in Poland), and their choice is limited. In Portugal, waiting lists for home care are longer in villages than in cities. In some countries (e.g. Bulgaria and Latvia) rehabilitation or specialized support (personal assistants, self-help organizations of people with disabilities, emergency calls, accessible housing, etc.) are available only in large cities. In other countries (particularly in the Czech Republic) competition between medical care and social care impairs the home-care infrastructure – regions with well developed medical facilities and services do not have a dense network of home care and vice versa. In Scandinavian countries, as well as Latvia and Slovenia, municipalities are responsible for collecting a large part of the funds for home care. As a consequence, rural communities with a high percentage of older individuals face problems covering just the need for care.

3.3.6 Evaluating access to home care

Selected aspects of access and accessibility have been analysed in this section. Despite this selective approach, it becomes clear that the principle "home care for all in need" has not been realized. In many countries, access to services is driven by available funding rather than needs. Conditions are relatively quite good in the Scandinavian countries. In Austria, Belgium, England, France, Ireland, Luxembourg and the Netherlands, individuals are eligible for a large variety of services too. However, long-term funding is becoming a problem in these countries. A huge variety of factors restricts access and accessibility elsewhere in Europe. Unmet needs – differences between needs and actually accessible care – were highest in Bulgaria, Croatia, Cyprus, Greece and Romania. Access to personal assistance or support for social activities is particularly restricted. These are among those services that are not covered by social insurance or the public budget and have to be purchased on the commercial market in many countries.

3.4 Informal caregivers and their role in the care process

In the majority of EU countries, informal caregivers provide a great deal of the care needed, estimated at 60% of the total, on average. In Greece, 90% of care is provided by families (Eurofamcare, 2006). The same situation exists in some central European countries. In contrast, only 15% of the care tasks are performed by family members in Denmark (Eurofamcare, 2006). People who are already users of formal services also receive a large amount of informal care from their families. According to the European Ad HOC study completed in 11 countries, informal caregivers provide a large portion of complementary care. The *median* number of hours of informal care per week ranged from 28 hours in Italy and 21 hours in France to 'only' 2 hours in Finland and Denmark and 0 hours in Sweden (Garms-Homolová, 2008). These variations may be explained by the availability of formal services and the general population's attitude towards the role of informal caregivers. The latter explanation translates into the family's moral and legal responsibility to care for its elderly members.

The general population's attitude towards the role of informal caregivers may also determine the way in which home-care services are organized. The historical background of the state's legal responsibility for its citizens is equally important. A family has no legal responsibilities for dependent members in Scandinavian countries because local authorities are explicitly responsible for care provision and reimbursement. The same holds for more market-oriented countries such as England, Luxembourg and Switzerland.

The issue of whether informal care substitutes or complements formal service remains open. In some countries (as in Bulgaria and Romania), informal caregivers are almost the only ones caring for disabled family members at home. The formal divide of responsibilities for caring varies in eastern European countries that have started to develop their formal services in the last two decades. The Scandinavian countries and the Netherlands provide fewer hours of informal care in comparison to the other countries because dense networks of efficiently working services are available.

3.4.1 Formal services taking available informal care into account

In England or Denmark, for instance, legislation takes the role of informal caregivers into account and assessment of their needs is obligatory. Ten countries[9] in this study follow another way of 'officially' recognizing the role of informal caregivers – regulation requires the availability of the informal system to be taken into consideration when their services decide on the allocation of care. This is particularly true in the allocation of services compensating for IADL dependency. However, many countries usually take these into account implicitly – by taking the availability of informal carers into account when assigning services. In about half of these countries, the availability of informal caregivers was a determining factor in the allocation of help with basic ADL. Other countries show huge differences between municipalities and therefore the experts interviewed in the EURHOMAP study were unable to estimate the importance of the availability of informal care for decisions on eligibility. However, even in countries where entitlement to home care is deemed only needs based (as in France), the care plan usually takes account of the contribution of informal caregivers, depending on the local authority. In some countries, efforts are in place to increase families' responsibilities through financial reimbursement of their contribution to care (as in Austria and Germany).

3.4.2 Informal versus formal caregivers: a new blurred frontier

Before the 1990s, informal caregivers were characterized as people with no training for care and as people who were ready to spend unlimited time on care. They were seen as permanently 'on duty' and as helpers who asked neither for contracts legalizing their responsibilities nor for payment or social security entitlement. The EURHOMAP data show that this perception continues in some countries. In the majority of eastern European and Mediterranean countries, the contribution of informal caregivers represents a resource that is taken for granted (compare Twigg & Atkin, 1994). But, increasingly, training is provided to informal caregivers in some countries (e.g. Belgium). Other countries provide informal caregivers with some reimbursement for their work or the chance of respite care (see Section 2.3). In England, informal caregivers are entitled to specific social benefits only if they are not related to the care receiver. In Austria and the Czech Republic, social benefits are available for family members who act as caregivers.

---

9 Belgium, Bulgaria, Greece, Italy, the Netherlands, Poland, Portugal, Romania, Slovakia and Slovenia.

Recent studies indicate that informal care has become "formalized" in the course of the last 15 years (Ungerson & Yeandle, 2007; Da Roit, Le Bihan & Öesterle, 2007; Burau, Theobald & Blank, 2007). The distinction between informal and formal care has become blurred because informal caregivers increasingly are paid for care and are obliged to collaborate with professionals. The introduction of direct payments or cash benefits (see Section 3.3) and the existence of various payment schemes enable clients to hire and pay caregivers according to their perceived needs.

Throughout Europe, the concepts and implementation of direct payment appear to differ according to:

- entitlement rules, number and type of beneficiaries;
- target group (either client or the informal caregiver);
- amount of money (compared to benefits in kind) and the social rights linked to it;
- procedure for testing eligibility and specific use during utilization and for assessing the quality of services provided; and
- whether only cash benefits are available or there is a choice between benefits in kind or in cash (as in England, France, Germany and Sweden).[10]

Several difficulties are attached to attendance allowance schemes. In France, cash benefits through the care attendance allowance scheme (*allocation personalisée d'autonomie*) are the backbone of public support for home care. However, benefits in kind remain the preferred option for users. Direct payments, subject to a lower level of control, are used by about 9% of the beneficiaries who hire informal caregivers. This difference in monitoring raises questions about the differences in the quality of provided services. In times of unemployment and economic uncertainty there is a risk that families could use the money for purposes other than buying care, as discussed by experts from Germany and Austria. This is also an issue related to the employment of migrant workers on the basis of cash benefits.

In a number of countries (e.g. the Netherlands, Norway, Slovenia and Sweden) formal contracts define informal carers' responsibilities and duties as well as the duration of the working time. Still, our data indicate that informal caregivers are paid less than formal caregivers in most of those countries in which direct payments were introduced. Similarly, their working conditions and entitlement to social rights are less favourable than those of formal caregivers. Some country experts assumed that the direct payment is not intended to support informal

---

10 In France, the amount of care is equal for both types of benefit. In Germany, benefits in kind guarantee a higher level of care provision than cash benefits.

caregivers but rather to limit the provision of formal care and reduce spending on long-term care. Supporting informal caregivers as 'co-workers' (Glendinning & Kemp, 2008) helps to secure the continuity of care because informal caregivers and family members are always 'available'. However, the efficacy of such an arrangement depends not only on the extent and type of coordination and integration between informal and formal caregivers, but also (and much more) on the availability of a sufficient workforce of formal caregivers. In a number of countries (e.g. the Netherlands, Norway, Slovenia, Sweden and, to some extent, in Italy) formal regulations define informal caregivers' responsibilities and duties as well as the duration of their working hours.

Finally, with the introduction of cash benefits or direct payments, family members who have gained new responsibilities for caring for their ill and disabled relatives sometimes experience deterioration in their health and social isolation. As a consequence, informal caregivers are considered clients of supporting services in many countries (i.e. they have needs resulting from their caring tasks) (Twigg & Atkin, 1994). This is the case in England, for instance, where caregivers' needs are assessed and supported through respite care. As shown in Chapter 2 (Section 2.3), public funding of respite care services is not common although counselling of family caregivers is publicly funded in many countries. The EURHOMAP data show that support for informal caregivers is associated with less developed formal services. But there is still a need to provide an adequate level of care overall and to seek to ensure quality of services. The ability to provide a reasonable amount of formal services remains the major requirement for such an achievement.

3.5 Challenges and developments

In most European countries, people prefer to receive care in their homes rather than in long-term care institutions. Only a minority of Europeans wish to move to a long-term care facility and the policies in Europe clearly encourage home-care arrangements as they are considered more cost efficient.

Our study showed that home-care infrastructure and provision is available to at least some extent in all European countries. All countries have created a financial basis that enables their citizens to use at least some forms of services. National experts were asked about unmet needs in their country. Relatively few were identified in Denmark, Finland, Luxembourg, the Netherlands and Norway. Various unmet needs were found in all other countries. In particular, some groups of the population face greater difficulties in accessing home services, and certain types of services are underrepresented in individual countries or regions within the countries. Often, it is easy to get physical care and help but difficult to get psychological support and psychosocial care. The reason may be eligibility and financial coverage but also differences in the availability of informal carers. Poor countries have poor services. This is true in terms of the low density of (qualified) home-care services; limited information on how to access them; and limited choice between different providers and types of care. Deficits in formal care are compensated by informal caregivers. However, the division of tasks between the formal and informal system depends on cultural values, the composition of families and attitudes to older members of society too (i.e. the importance of autonomy).

Information on unmet needs is not collected systematically in most countries. As a result, this will not find its way easily onto national policy agendas and policy options may be difficult to formulate when it does. The existing research focuses on few aspects of the complex problem of access and accessibility. As a consequence, few data are available and it is difficult to draw a real comparison across countries and types of care users. Nonetheless, some countries are very active in measuring not only needs but also factors determining access to care – for example, Ireland (Delaney, 2009) and the Netherlands (Algera, 2005). One main subject in future discussions on home care will be how to prevent (unmet) needs through the best mix of extending or tailoring formal care, self care, informal care and support for, and use of, technology.

The EURHOMAP study has identified the following topics for policy-makers' attention:

- Inequalities in access to home care are considerable across Europe. Policy-makers may need to make efforts to reduce them.
- Client relations management is required (e.g. development of: easy and accessible information; communication between payers, services and clients; care management; and counselling). Also, greater empowerment of clients and their relatives. In this regard, the potential impact of growing commercialization concerning access to and the quality of home care, and client empowerment, will become an important topic for research.
- Integration of social services and health care on all levels (policy, eligibility, provision, reimbursement, quality control), particularly the integration of home care and home nursing, is an indispensable condition for optimal services.
- Continuous adjustment of benefits to actual needs will be required in most countries.

At present, informal care is preferred to professional care in many countries (e.g. in southern or south-east Europe) but, even there, family care and other informal care is expected to decline and old-age dependency ratios are increasing. This chapter has discussed different forms of support for informal caregivers and shown the need for new reservoirs of informal care. Efforts to increase the visibility of unmet needs could motivate potential volunteers and intensify informal engagement in caring for and helping people in need. Care provided outside the registers (often by immigrant workers in some countries) may also become a future policy issue. In any case, policy-makers need to find solutions to the mistreatment of immigrant workers (i.e. unfair wages, social security and working conditions) and to safeguard the quality of care of such unregistered providers. As its importance grows, policy-makers may need to consider legalizing and formalizing such types of informal care (as in Austria, Cyprus and Italy).

Overall, the empowerment of home-care recipients and their families will be an important goal of future home-care policies. Informal carers will certainly continue to be major contributors to home care. Safeguarding the pool of informal caregivers will therefore become one of the main challenges for future governments. The central issue is whether informal caregivers' contributions will take place on the basis of their real choice (which frequently corresponds to older people's expectations). Governments will need to achieve a balance between three options. First, extensive use of informal caregivers would reduce long-term care budgets. However, this is only a short-term solution. The data show that a better option would be to establish the best balance between informal and formal carers. This could be achieved by securing measures that have proved efficient in enabling potential carers within the labour market to work while caring. It would also be necessary to maintain (or extend) professional services as care needs for the older population continue to grow. Another option would be to introduce measures (e.g. training and respite care) which would allow older carers to continue to care for an extended period of their longer life in good conditions. A further option would be to promote healthy ageing and social integration, leading to enhanced social capital. In turn, this might contribute to reduced future care needs and help solve the supply side issue by offering more opportunity for volunteers to contribute to the older care sector.

References

Algera M (2005). *All you need is ... home care. Matches between home care needed, indicated and delivered; a study among chronic patients.* Utrecht, Netherlands Institute for Health Services Research (http://www.nivel.nl/sites/default/files/

bestanden/All-you-need-is-home-care-proefschrift-2005.pdf, accessed 24 August 2012).

Bonsang E (2009). Does informal care from children to their elderly parents substitute for formal care in Europe? *Journal of Health Economics* 28(1):143–154.

Burau V, Theobald H, Blank R (2007). *Governing home care: a cross national comparison.* Cheltenham, Edward Elgar Publishing.

Da Roit B, Le Bihan B, Öesterle A (2007). Long-term care policies in Italy, Austria and France: variations in cash-for-care schemes. *Social Policy & Administration*, 41(6):653–671.

Delaney L et al. (2009). *SHARE Ireland – survey of health, ageing and retirement in Europe.* Dublin, University College Dublin Geary Institute.

Eurofamcare (2006). *The trans-European survey report (TEUSURE).* Hamburg, Services for Supporting Family Carers of Elderly People in Europe: Characteristics, Coverage & Usage (http://www.uke.de/extern/eurofamcare/deli.php, accessed 5 June 2012).

Garms-Homolovà V (2008). Koproduktion in häuslicher Pflege – Informelle Hilfe für Empfänger berufsmäßiger Pflege in elf europäischen Ländern: Die Ad HOC – Studie. In: Zank S, Hedke-Becker A, eds. *Generationen in Familie und Gesellschaft im demographischen Wandel. Europäische Perspektiven.* Stuttgart, Kohlhammer:146–164.

Genre V, Salvador RG, Lamo A (2011). *European women – why do(n't) they work?* Frankfurt, European Central Bank.

Glendinning C, Kemp PA, eds. (2008). *Cash and care; policy challenges in the welfare state.* Bristol, The Policy Press.

Gulliford M, Figueroa-Munoz J, Morgan M (2003). Introduction: measuring of 'access' in health care. In: Gulliford M, Myfanwy M, eds. *Access to health care.* London, Routledge:1–12.

Millmann ML (1993). *Access to health care in America.* Washington, DC, Institute of Medicine, National Academy Press.

OECD (2010). OECD Health Data [offline database]. *Services of long-term nursing care.* Paris, Organisation for Economic Co-operation and Development (http://www.oecd.org/health/, accessed June 2010).

Penchansky R, Thomas JW (1981). The concept of access: a definition and relationship to consumer satisfaction. *Medical Care*, 19(2):127–140.

SHARE (2009). *Survey of Health, Ageing and Retirement in Europe (SHARE). Release 2.3.1 – Wave 2.* Munich (http://share-dev.mpisoc.mpg.de/home.html, accessed 5 June 2012).

TNS Opinion & Social (2007). Health and long-term care in the European Union. Brussels, European Commission, *Special Eurobarometer 283/Wave 67.3.*

Twigg J, Atkin K (1994). *Carers perceived: policy and practice in informal care.* Buckingham, Open University Press.

Ungerson CL, Yeandle S, eds. (2007). *Cash for care in developed welfare states.* Basingstoke, Palgrave MacMillan.

Viitanen TK (2005). *Informal elderly care and female labour force participation across Europe.* Brussels, European Network of Economic Policy Research Institutes (ENEPRI Research Report No.13).

Chapter 4
Management of the care process

Nadine Genet, Allen Hutchinson, Michel Naiditch, Vjenka Garms-Homolovà, Cecilia Fagerström, Maria Gabriella Melchiorre, Madelon Kroneman, Cosetta Greco

4.1 Introduction

Management of the care process refers to the actual provision of home care. The comprehensiveness of services delivered in clients' homes appears to vary widely across Europe – for example, regarding the number of publicly funded home-care services, the average number of hours of home care provided and the proportion of the population receiving home care. Alongside different levels of informal care there are inter-country differences in the organization, availability, accessibility and quality of the care process; together with issues such as the coordination of service delivery, competition in delivery and methods by which the quality of services is safeguarded in each country. Since the organization of home care is currently in significant transition in many countries, implementation problems may also influence home-care provision.

This chapter will explore characteristics of the care process in practice. Thus, the focus will be on the organization of actual provision of home care and will address the following aspects – types of provider; competition between providers; integration of care; human resources; and quality of care. The chapter will conclude with an overview of the challenges and current concerns in home-care delivery.

4.2 Who provides home care?

This section explores two important features of home-care provision: (i) the ownership of providers of services; and (ii) the extent to which there is competition among providers.

Broadly, there are two types of ownership for home-care providers – publicly and privately owned organizations. Publicly owned providers fall under the direct control of government (at national, regional or local level) and thus can be directly influenced by it. Privately owned organizations cannot be influenced so directly and therefore other forms of steering are required, for example, to ensure quality and to determine the means of price setting. A further distinction must also be made between privately owned providers who are funded publicly and privately owned providers who are hired by the client directly, without public resources.

When public resources are used to commission services from privately owned providers, these providers can be influenced by, for instance, compulsory contracts with (local) governments. When more than one provider is available, competition may also play a role. Competition may be used to enhance the quality and efficiency of home-care provision or competition may lead to more choice, either for clients (who can choose from which provider they wish to receive care) or for governments (who can choose which provider to contract). Whether and how competition exists depends on the national or regional policy and regulatory framework, as well as the type of organizations that provide home care.

Our results show that publicly owned providers are the most prevalent provider type. However, there are many different types of public provider across countries. For example, there are municipalities providing health and social care (as in the Scandinavian countries) or only social home care (as in Slovenia). There are national health service agencies (as in England); municipal or regional state agencies for social services (as in Greece and Bulgaria); and semi-state-owned organizations (as in Bulgaria). In some countries, negative incentives that may arise when public organizations are both funder and provider of services are counteracted by disentangling these two functions. In several Scandinavian countries, there may be separate departments in a municipality – those that provide the services and those that are responsible for the budget. This system is meant to create pressures for efficiency on the provider units. In some Finnish municipalities these units may compete with privately owned organizations offering household services.

For private providers, a distinction needs to be made between non-profit-making and profit-making providers. In some countries the non-profit-making sector is extensive and comprises a mix of voluntary, charitable and professionally led organizations. This sector may involve many different organizations – for example, there are charitable organizations (e.g. in Bulgaria and England), some with church affiliations. Further examples include voluntary organizations (volunteers, sometimes mixed with professionals); small professional teams; or, sometimes, large professional non-profit-making organizations. Some of these large non-profit-making organizations were previously charitable organizations (e.g. in Luxembourg and the Netherlands).

Each type of organization may affect costs, accessibility and quality of care differently. Profit-making organizations usually face the rigours of the market place but this may also apply to non-profit-making organizations. Both types of privately owned providers can work in a wide range of settings, for example:

- directly publicly funded and regulated settings in which private contracted home care agencies (e.g. in the Netherlands) or private individuals are funded directly by governments or through social insurance;

- indirectly funded and regulated settings in which private home-care agencies are funded through vouchers (e.g. in Belgium) or where private home-care agencies (e.g. in Finland) or individuals (e.g. in Cyprus and Austria) are funded by clients – whether or not they receive benefits from the government or social insurance, they may be registered and subject to inspections (e.g. in Finland); and

- privately funded and lightly regulated settings (some regions in Italy).

Most of the information available on non-profit-making and profit-making providers relates to those providers funded by public money, with relatively little information available about private resources being spent on care in these sectors. Hence, although evidence from some experts suggests that private clients pay considerable sums of money for home care, this study has not been able to provide a complete overview of all parts of the 'private sector'.

In most countries there is a mixed economy of home-care provision – that is, privately owned providers (profit-making and non-profit-making) provide home nursing care and social home care alongside public providers (see Table 4.1). Often, the main type of provider in home nursing is also the main type in social home care, but in eastern European countries the main type of home nursing provider is more likely to be private and profit-making than is the social home-care provider. The involvement of privately owned providers seems to be increasing in several countries (e.g. Belgium, Croatia, Denmark, Finland, Iceland and Sweden). Profit-making provision is growing in France. In these countries, home care is increasingly seen as a 'profitable business'. Such profit-making organizations are filling the gaps that may result from limited availability or limited accessibility to the publicly funded and non-profit-making services and may be associated with higher quality and better accessibility. For example, in Ireland the (limited) provision of an integrated service day and night, seven days a week, is mainly provided by the private sector. Simultaneously, shortages in private home-care agencies were reported in some countries (e.g. Latvia).

Table 4.1 Ownership of home-care providers and the existence of competition in 31 European countries

Country	Main type of provider (x) h = home health care s = social home care			Other important types of provider (x) h = home health care s = social home care			Competition X = exists P = partly Empty = no competition[a]	Extent to which a home-care market exists
	Publicly owned	Privately owned non-profit-making	Privately owned profit-making	Publicly owned	Privately owned non-profit-making	Privately owned profit-making		
Austria		X		X				Low
Belgium		X		Xs		Xh	X	High
Bulgaria	Xs	Xh	Xh		X	Xh		High
Croatia	X	Xs		Xs	X	Xh		Medium
Cyprus	X				X	X		Low
Czech Republic	Xs	X	X		Xs			Low
Denmark	X					X		Low
England			X	X	X		X	High
Estonia	Xs		Xh	Xh	Xs	Xs	X	High
Finland	X				Xs	Xs		Low
France		X		Xs	X	X	X	High
Germany		X	X	X	X	X	X	High
Greece	Xs		Xh	Xh	X			Medium
Hungary	X				Xh		P	Low
Iceland	X				Xs	Xh		Low
Ireland	X				X	X	X	Medium
Italy	Xhs	Xs				X	X	Medium
Latvia	X				Xs	Xh		Low
Lithuania	X				X	Xs		Low
Luxembourg		X				X	X	High

Table 4.1 contd

Country	Main type of provider (x) h = home health care s = social home care			Other important types of provider (x) h = home health care s = social home care			Competition X = exists P = partly Empty = no competition[a]	Extent to which a home-care market exists
	Publicly owned	Privately owned non-profit-making	Privately owned profit-making	Publicly owned	Privately owned non-profit-making	Privately owned profit-making		
Malta	Xs	Xh				X		Medium
Netherlands		X				X	X	High
Norway	X				X			Low
Poland	Xs		Xh	Xh		Xs		High
Portugal	Xh	Xs			Xh	X	P	Medium
Romania	X				X	X		Low
Slovakia	Xs	Xh			Xs	Xs		Medium
Slovenia	X				X	Xs		Low
Spain	Xs	Xh		Xh	Xs	Xs	P	Medium
Sweden	X				Xs		X	Medium
Switzerland	X				X			Low

[a] X: Several providers and competition possible; P: Partly: competition in one area of home care; Empty box: monopoly or several providers but in practice no competition.

In these countries, the private sector does not seem to be interested in entering the home-care market since this is not considered to be profitable. The lack of interest of individuals and organizations seems to be partially responsible for the shortages in home-care provision in these countries.

Competition seems to exist to some extent in at least 14 countries. Although providers are increasing in type and number, real competition is still absent in most countries. Even if there is free choice of provider in theory, competition remains absent due to a shortage of home-care providers. Moreover, in many countries there is only one provider in one area. In general, marketization of home care seems highest in Belgium, England, France, Germany, Luxembourg and the Netherlands, where private providers of either type (sometimes alongside public providers) are involved in publicly financed home care.

4.3 Integrated home-care delivery

Integration of home-care services is important to prevent overlap or gaps in service provision and thus it may enhance quality and efficiency. According to Grilz-Wolf et al. (2004), integration consists of "linking parts within a single level of care, for instance the creation of multiprofessional teams (horizontal integration) or the linking between different levels of care, i.e. primary, secondary and tertiary care (vertical integration)". Therefore, two types of integration are applicable to home care: (i) integration within the different home-care services; and (ii) integration between home-care services and other care sectors. Ways of integration in practice will be presented throughout this section, with reference to innovative practices[1] that were mentioned by country experts throughout Europe.

4.3.1 Integrated delivery of home-care services

Integrated delivery of home-care services can be attained in, broadly, three main ways (Table 4.2). The first is organizational integration, in which *one organization* or team provides all types of home-care services. Where it works well, it is characterized by clear task differentiation for professionals and clear access points for patients (Table 4.2). The second, the *coordinator* model, seeks to coordinate home-care services provided by different organizations through case managers; through other structural links between home-care professionals from different organizations; or through the formulation of individual care

---

[1] In the EURHOMAP study experts were asked to mention innovative practices for their country related to home care. No knowledge of home care in other countries was required for an innovation to be identified. Almost all were meant to enhance the delivery and accessibility of home care. We present some of these innovative practices in the following pages. Descriptions of these innovative practices can be found on www.nivel.eu/eurhomap. It is also important to note that the selection criteria for these innovative practices may have excluded new and valuable ideas from this discussion.

Table 4.2 *Models of integration for home health and social home care*

One organization	Coordinator	Voluntary
Features		
• organizations and teams providing both home nursing care and social home care	• home-care organizations mainly provide either home nursing, or personal care or domestic aid	• home-care providers mainly provide only one type of home care
• good integration of services	• integrated assessment of needs	• professionals themselves decide when to contact other professionals
• clear task differentiation between professionals	• home care is coordinated through a multidisciplinary care plan	• professionals have no clear task differentiation
• clear access		
However, such cases may still have specialized services that are not integrated. For instance, care that is provided after surgery only; service provides care only to children; or service is provided only to people who need percutaneous endoscopic gastrostomy (PEG) or tube feeding etc.	• a coordinator is in charge of the care plan (may be assessor), either an individual or a special organization	
	• clear task division between professionals for certain types of case or in individual care process	
	• often found for 'complex' home-care patients (in need of multidisciplinary care)	
	• a coordinator may be assigned to special cases and meetings will be held with all professionals involved	

plans. Either a coordinator is assigned (possibly only in the assessment phase) or regular meetings take place on complex cases. Home care can be coordinated through a multidisciplinary care plan, based on an integrated assessment of needs and a clear task division between professionals in an individual care process (Table 4.2). The third model is integration on a *voluntary* basis. In this case, professionals themselves decide when to contact other professionals and there is no clear task differentiation among the different professionals (Table 4.2).

Many new initiatives have recently been set up to improve organizational integration. Their functions are often reflected in their names – for example, the multipurpose services of help and care at home (Services Polyvalents d'Aide et de Soins à Domicile) in France, home-care centres in Finland or integrated home help (Assistenza Domiciliare Integrata – ADI) in Italy. In the Netherlands, small-scale neighbourhood teams of home-care professionals (known as neighbourhood care) are competing increasingly with large-scale providers. These teams were set up as a reaction to the scaling-up of home

Table 4.3 *Integration of home-care delivery throughout Europe*

Country	Strength of organizational integration • = segregated •• = partly integrated ••• = integrated [a]	Strength of formal coordination • = hardly anywhere •• = in some areas ••• = usually
Austria	•	••
Belgium (Wallonia/Flanders)	•• •	••
Bulgaria	•• •	•
Croatia [b]	••	••
Cyprus	•	•
Czech Republic	•••	•
Denmark	•••	•••
England	•	•••
Estonia	•	•
Finland	••	•••
France	••	•
Germany	•••	••
Greece	••	••
Hungary	•	•
Iceland	••	•••
Ireland	••	•••
Italy	••	••
Latvia	•	•
Lithuania	•	•
Luxembourg	•••	•••
Malta	•	••
Netherlands	••	•••
Norway	•••	•••
Poland	••	••
Portugal	••	•
Romania	N/A	N/A
Slovakia	•	•
Slovenia	•	•
Spain	•	•
Sweden	••	•••
Switzerland [b]	••	• •••

[a] • Almost always segregated (integration very rare); •• significant (but not main) part integrated; ••• integrated – (almost) all providers providing all service. [b] Integration of personal care and nursing at home. However, domestic aid is provided separately by NGOs (but this service is scarce).

care and the resulting disintegration of home-care delivery. It is said that the teams have increased efficiency and the quality of service provision (they score highest on patient satisfaction). In the Netherlands, the At Home with Dementia project established an even wider interdisciplinary care chain to treat, support and advise people with dementia and their families. In many countries coordination is not actually structural, but rather depends on the willingness of the professionals and agencies involved, as in the voluntary model.

In practice the coordinator model takes several forms across Europe. There can be coordination only at the start (see also Chapter 3) or during the whole period of service provision. Additionally, coordination of care can be the responsibility of one person, a team or a whole organization; and/or a written plan can be used.

Where one professional is responsible for the coordination of care, it is usually a social worker, nurse or GP. For instance, GPs are coordinators in Latvia and Slovakia – in the former they are legally responsible. Social workers are coordinators in four countries;[2] nurses in four countries;[3] and special case managers are responsible in seven countries.[4] Organizations with special responsibility for home care-coordination exist in some countries – for example, the Integrated Services for Home Care (Geïntegreerde Dienst voor Thuisverzorging or Service Intégré de Soins à Domicile) in Belgium. These organize multidisciplinary consultations of primary health-care and social home-care professionals and support the development of multidisciplinary care plans. Additionally, home-care centres and care managers of sickness funds offer support and information for all professionals, as well as the client. Long-term care support centres (Pflegestützpunkte) with case managers to inform clients about available services are being introduced in Germany. Sometimes, such counselling services are provided by the long-term care insurance funds but more often they are the responsibility of the community or a charity. The Italian geriatric evaluation units (Unità Valutativa Geriatrica) set up care plans for elderly people and monitor subsequent needs.

Personal plans can be used to set tasks and their coordination; these are common in many countries[5] and take many forms. For example, ADI in Italy uses a multidisciplinary assessment at home to produce a personal care plan and a linked individualized budget. In Norway, there is a legal obligation for the services involved in the care of younger people to establish an individual plan. However, utilization is low, even among those population groups who are in need, and personal plans are seldom used for elderly people despite the need.

There are many examples of coordinating arrangements across Europe. Often, these formal coordinating arrangements pertain mainly to people with complex needs. Examples include integrated care for people with dementia in Austria; case managers for young people with severe disabilities or people with severe

---

2 Belgium, Greece, Ireland and Lithuania.
3 Denmark, Ireland, the Netherlands and Norway.
4 Denmark, England, Iceland, Ireland, Norway and in some specific cases in France and Portugal.
5 For example, France, Italy, Luxembourg, the Netherlands, Norway and in some Finnish municipalities and some cases in Belgium.

Alzheimer disease in France; or people with complex clinical and social needs in Ireland.

The level of coordination of formal care seems lowest in the Baltic States, Bulgaria, Cyprus, France, Italy, Portugal, Slovakia, Slovenia and Spain (Table 4.3). Additionally, there are intra-country differences, either because there is a scarcity of appropriate professionals in some areas and organizations or because, as in Iceland, the remoteness of rural areas makes it difficult to coordinate home health care with home social care. The coordination between publicly and privately owned organizations will become an important issue as the number of private providers grows. For instance, in Finland health information systems used by all home-care and other care providers are accessible only for public providers. However, there is already cooperation between private and public providers in a number of countries (e.g. Austria, Cyprus, England and Italy).

Coordination of care by GPs and home-care providers

Overall, the level of formal coordination between GPs and home care strongly depends on the type of home care – coordination with home health care is stronger, as would be expected (see Table 4.4). Many governments (e.g. in Austria and the Netherlands) are trying to improve coordination between GPs and home care. Coordination takes place through a number of routes. The GP can be a formal referral agent – they are the exclusive gatekeepers for some types of home nursing in eleven countries,[6] and one of the two possible referral agents in two other countries.[7] In some countries, the GP also sets up a care plan (as in Bulgaria) or is responsible for the coordination of care (as in Latvia and in complex cases in Finland).

Another route towards coordination – working together in teams/small organizations – occurs in ten countries.[8] For example, teams of community care professionals that include a GP and a social worker provide integrated home care for adults in some areas of Ireland. In England and the Netherlands these teams are based in the same buildings.

In another, rarer, route formal agreements are established between home-care providers and GPs. One example of such 'institutionalized' coordination is the funding of Belgium's Cooperation Initiatives in Primary Health Care (Samenwerkingsinitiatieven Eerstelijnsgezondheidszorg). These are aimed at safeguarding the quality of care and the cooperation between professionals. Another example is the national primary care agreements/guidelines for cooperation and task differentiation for specific types of care (Landelijke

---

[6] Belgium, Bulgaria, Estonia, Germany, Latvia, Malta, Romania, Slovenia; Czech Republic and Poland (where it is only necessary for financing of home nursing); Iceland (for social care).
[7] In Lithuania (other is social worker) and Sweden (other is community nurse).
[8] England, Ireland, Latvia, Lithuania, Malta, the Netherlands, Poland, Portugal, Slovenia and Spain.

Table 4.4 Integration of home-care delivery with other types of care

Country	Coordination with GPs[a] • = absent •• = selected cases ••• = structural (H= home health care, S= social home care)	Coordination with hospital • = hardly anywhere •• = in some areas ••• = usually (H= home health care, S= social home care)	Coordination with nursing homes/ residential care • = hardly anywhere •• = in some areas ••• = usually (H= home health care, S= social home care)
Austria	••	•	•
Belgium	••	•••	•
Bulgaria	•	•	•
Croatia	••• (H) N/A (S)	•	• N/A (S)
Cyprus	••	•	• (H) ••• (S)
Czech Republic	••	•	•
Denmark	••• (H) •• (S)	•••	••
England	••	•••	••
Estonia	••• (H) • (S)	•••	•
Finland	•••	•••	•••
France	•	•	•
Germany	•••	•••	••
Greece	•	•	N/A
Hungary	••• (H) • (S)	••	••
Iceland	••	•	•
Ireland	••	••	•
Italy	••• (H) • (S)	••	••
Latvia	••• (H) • (S)	•••	•
Lithuania	•• (H) • (S)	•	•••
Luxembourg	••	••	••
Malta	••• (H) • (S)	••• (H) • (S)	••
Netherlands	••	•••	•••
Norway	•	•••	••
Poland	••• (H) • (S)	••	•
Portugal	••	••	N/A
Romania	N/A	•	•
Slovakia	••• (H) • (S)	••	•••
Slovenia	•• •	••	• •••

[a] • Formal coordination between GPs and home care was absent, present in very few areas or GPs acted only as formal referral agents for special technical nursing cases; •• only in specific patient cases; ••• formal coordination was presented as strong when home health care and general practices were usually organizationally integrated or there were often agreements on cooperation between the two and if they are a formal referral agent for home care. N/A: no information available.

Table 4.4 *contd*

Country	Coordination with <u>GPs</u>[a] • = absent •• = selected cases ••• = structural (H= home health care, S= social home care)	Coordination with <u>hospital</u> • = hardly anywhere •• = in some areas ••• = usually (H= home health care, S= social home care)	Coordination with nursing homes/ residential care • = hardly anywhere •• = in some areas ••• = usually (H= home health care, S= social home care)
Spain	•• (H) •(S)	•••	••
Sweden	•••	•••	•••
Switzerland	••	•	•

[a] • Formal coordination between GPs and home care was absent, present in very few areas or GPs acted only as formal referral agents for special technical nursing cases; •• only in specific patient cases; ••• formal coordination was presented as strong when home health care and general practices were usually organizationally integrated or there were often agreements on cooperation between the two and if they are a formal referral agent for home care. N/A: no information available.

Eerstelijns Samenwerkings Afspraken) in the Netherlands. These lay down agreements concerning diagnosis, care provider and care provision and coordination for several conditions.

Coordination through cooperation guidelines is not yet widespread because existing guidelines were often developed for specific types of care within health-care provision only (e.g. palliative and dementia care as in Austria, the Netherlands and Poland). Additionally, the role of coordinator can be taken by a nurse (e.g. as in Belgium, Luxembourg and the Netherlands) or a home-care worker. The latter may (even) have formal responsibilities to accompany a client to the GP or to notify the doctor if the client's health deteriorates (as in Bulgaria and the Czech Republic).

4.3.2 Coordination between hospitals and home-care providers

Coordination between hospitals and home-care providers may take place in two different situations. First, home care may be necessary after hospital discharge – hospitals and home-care providers may cooperate to enable a smooth transition and continuity of care. Secondly, hospitals may cooperate with home care to prevent hospital admission, either by enabling patients to remain at home – even in cases where the patient's condition would normally require hospitalization – or to shorten hospital admission by enabling the patient to recover further at home (e.g. through rehabilitation at home).

Coordination between home health care and hospital care in the case of hospital discharge is relatively strong in Europe, taking place mainly through liaison nurses working for either the hospital or the home-care organization involved. Social workers may also be responsible for organizing home care after discharge, and for social home-care services. In Finland, uniform electronic patient records are accessible to hospitals and home-care providers. This also enables a municipality to see when patients are to be discharged and make necessary arrangements. Other networks involve case managers for complex cases. A law in Germany includes passages concerning coordination during discharge from hospital to home care (see country report).

Examples of the integration of home care and hospital care can be found in several countries. The integrated home care and discharge practice for home-care clients (PALKO model) in Finland included activities to safeguard continuity, especially between primary and specialized care, such as supporting the coping process of elderly people being discharged to home and involving a home-nurse/home-helper pairing in discharge planning at the hospital. In England, structured hospital systems have been developed to assess care needs after discharge at an early stage. These result in a 're-ablement' package for up to six weeks after discharge, either in the home or in an intermediate care facility in the community. Some hospitals provide (specialized) home health care (as in Italy, Latvia and Spain). Coordinated pathways between hospital, primary care and social services have been set up in Denmark.

Hospitalization at home, as an alternative to inpatient admission, is a growing sector in France and Spain. This is seen as a cheaper alternative to inpatient care. Furthermore, it creates the possibility for patients to stay in the family environment (Afrite et al., 2007). Formal agreements between hospitals and municipalities have been set up in Norway. These require hospitals to provide professional guidance to home health-care professionals in order for them to acquire competence (e.g. in treatment of patients with a home ventilator).

In France, some multiprofessional geriatric networks in the Paris region are operating between the hospital and primary care sector. These are designed to help older people to stay in their own homes with only limited risk and/or avoiding unnecessary hospitalization. They focus on continuity of care between health care on the one hand and personal care and domestic aid on the other. The networks are run by a (usually hospital-based) physician with one or two coordinating nurses who act also as a liaison. Other networks involve case managers for complex cases.

4.3.3 Coordination between residential- and home-care providers

Generally, the coordination of home care and residential care is somewhat weaker across Europe than home care and hospital/GP care (see Table 4.4). Liaisons with regard to residential care were mentioned rarely by the experts interviewed in the study. Formal coordination takes place mainly on an organizational level rather than at a patient level. Some residential-care organizations do provide home care in some countries (e.g. in Scandinavian countries, Slovakia and in the Netherlands, about half of the home-care providers are also residential-care providers; in Spain, some private companies organize residential care and may have a specific division for home-care services). Still, at present this appears to be uncommon in Europe.

4.4 Human resources

Home care is a labour-intensive sector. Although some initiatives use modern technology to replace some human labour (for example, see Section 4.5 on telecare), home care is mainly a hands-on activity. The provision of home care that is quantitatively and qualitatively satisfactory requires workers who are available at the right time, the right place and with the right skills. Furthermore, quality and efficiency in home care may also be enhanced through effective human resource management methods.

Data on the number of home-care workers in any one country were not widely available to the review. Most was known about personal care providers – these showed the lowest densities in Croatia, the Czech Republic, Hungary and Latvia; and the highest in Denmark, Estonia, Italy, Norway and Sweden.

The growing number and proportion of elderly people, the declining workforce and the use of part-time workers in many countries may result in an increase in unmet needs in the near future. Experts in several countries spoke of their concerns about the shortage of qualified personnel. A general shortage of staff was reported in several countries,[9] as well as a lack of sufficiently qualified home care staff.[10] For instance, Belgium and Bulgaria have too few home helps; France, Greece, Lithuania and Slovenia have too few home-care professionals in general. Box 4.1 presents some innovative examples of dealing with shortages in human resources as reported by the country experts.

4.4.1 Different types of home-care worker

In all countries, professionally trained nurses are responsible for medically oriented technical tasks, prevention and therapeutic care. Social services are provided by a wide range of professionals, ranging from well trained social workers and personal social care workers to auxiliaries (domestic aid workers).

The widest range of home-care professionals exists in Norway, Belgium, Bulgaria and Romania (see Table 4.5). In many countries the tasks of professionals (especially those of nurses and personal carers) partially overlap. This is true in Belgium and France where they focus on different recipient groups, for example,

---

9 Austria, Belgium, Bulgaria, Cyprus, Czech Republic, Finland, France, Greece, Lithuania, Portugal and Slovenia.

10 Bulgaria, Cyprus, Denmark, Estonia, France, Germany, Greece, Luxembourg and Norway.

adults with disabilities and elderly people (France); people with complex disabilities and people with minor disabilities (Belgium). However, the borders of responsibility are not always clear. In Germany, the division of tasks between nurses and personal caregivers depends on the type of care provider. Private profit-making providers frequently deploy nurses for the entire spectrum of tasks because the division of labour would cause higher costs. Conversely, charitable organizations usually make a distinction between technical nursing that is reimbursed by the health-care funds, and long-term care (non-technical nursing) that is reimbursed by the long-term care insurance. While the first task is performed by nurses, the second is performed by less qualified caregivers.

Official national (or regional) task descriptions of home nurses exist in almost all countries. About half of the countries have laid down formal task descriptions for personal care; and just one third for domestic aid.

4.4.2 Educational level

All the countries under study have educational requirements for nurses. Generally, their training takes three to four years. In about one third of the countries, nurses require continuous recertification that involves additional training or passing a test every few years. Additional training was available in most countries but such recertification can be obtained voluntarily in many countries where recertification is not obligatory for nurses (e.g. Germany). Short additional courses are funded by the home-care agencies in just half the countries. Specialization (or postgraduate education) is possible in some countries – for example, for community nurses in Cyprus, England, Portugal and Sweden or nurse specialists in Belgium, Luxembourg and the Netherlands. However, in most countries, nurse specialists rarely work in home care.

In about 60% of the countries educational requirements exist for personal care professionals. However, the duration of the education varies much more than for home nursing – from three years in Spain to no qualification at all in Bulgaria and the Czech Republic. In several countries social workers are involved in home care, often as case managers. Most have a university degree with extensive postgraduate training.

People helping in the household also require some training in about one quarter of the countries. However, generally this is because they also provide personal care so training may pertain only to personal care. Only a minority of the domestic aid professionals were qualified in the Czech Republic, Poland and Romania. Additionally, there is uncertainty about whether requirements for qualification are being fulfilled in other countries (France, Greece and Hungary). Furthermore, home care requires only a very low level of basic schooling in

Greece, Malta and Portugal; and migrants from other countries provide a large share of home care in Austria, Cyprus and Italy. These migrants often do not have the required level of education and remain outside governmental regulatory control. However, this is changing in some countries. In Austria, for instance, these groups are being formalized (i.e. registered and assigned rights). While migration of staff can be valuable to some countries, this east–west migration can have a negative effect on human resources in eastern Europe and rural–urban migration may have a negative effect on human resources in rural areas.

4.4.3 Working conditions

Good working conditions are needed to recruit and retain qualified home-care workers. The following working conditions were investigated:

- whether tasks are laid down at national/regional level;
- whether home-care professionals have permanent working contracts;
- whether collective agreements on working conditions and salaries are in place; and
- home-care workers' salaries.

Working conditions differ greatly across types of profession (best for home-care nurses) but, generally, home-care workers tend to have a regular contract with a salary paid by a home-care agency or municipality. Most home-care professionals work in home care part-time. Self-employment is possible in most countries and is quite common (mainly for nurses) in Belgium, Estonia, France and Greece. Short-term contracts for social home-care workers are also common in several countries – in Greece and Lithuania these are the most usual type of contract. There is not much information about the salaries and contract status of social workers but our experts indicated that well trained social workers attract good salaries and have high educational levels.

Collective working condition agreements are quite common but often these hold only for professionals working in the *public* sector, or relate only to salaries and differ strongly between the home health-care and social home-care sectors.

4.4.4 Salaries

Among nurses, salaries tend to be best in Denmark and England, where they are above the average income, and relatively bad in Norway and Poland. Caution is needed when comparing the salaries of social home-care workers across countries as roles and tasks may differ widely (in some countries they also

Management of the care process **87**

Table 4.5 Indications for the quality of human resources

Country	Fragmentation of work			Quality standards			
	Types of professionals providing domestic aid No.	Types of professionals providing personal care No.	Types of professionals providing home nursing No.	Min. required educational level for professionals in:			Recertification of nurses required
				domestic aid[a]	personal care[b]	nursing[c]	
Austria	N/A	2	2	•	•	••	Yes
Belgium	2	6	4	•	•••	••	No
Bulgaria	4	4	1	•	•	•••	No
Croatia	N/A	3	N/A	•	N/A	N/A	N/A
Cyprus	3	3	2	••	••	•••	No
Czech Republic	N/A	3	1	••	••	•••	No
Denmark	2	2	2	•••	•••	•••	No
England	1	1	1	•	•	••	Yes
Estonia	1	3	1	••	•	•••	No
Finland	1	4	1	•	•••	•••	No
France	2	2	1	•	•	•••	No
Germany	3	2	2	••	••	•••	No
Greece	1	1	1	•	•	•••	No
Hungary	1	1	1	•	•	•••	Yes
Iceland	1	1	1	•	•	•••	No
Ireland	N/A	N/A	2	•	•	•••	No
Italy	2	2	1	••	•••	••	Yes
Latvia	3	3	2	••	••	•••	Yes
Lithuania	3	2	2	•	••	••	Yes
Luxembourg	2	3	2	•	•••	••	Yes

[a] • no education, •• short training by employer, ••• training longer than one month; [b] • 4 months or less, •• > 4 months, ••• > 6 months; [c] • 2 years or less, •• between 2 and 3 years, ••• > 3 years; N/A: no information available.

Table 4.5 contd

Country	Fragmentation of work			Quality standards			
	Types of professionals providing domestic aid No.	Types of professionals providing personal care No.	Types of professionals providing home nursing No.	Min. required educational level for professionals in:			Recertification of nurses required
				domestic aid[a]	personal care[b]	nursing[c]	
Malta	1	1	1	••	••	••	No
Netherlands	3	2	3	•	•••	••	Yes
Norway	3	7	3	••	•••	••	No
Poland	3	3	1	•••	•••	•••	Yes
Portugal	1	1	1	•	•	•••	No
Romania	4	4	N/A	N/A	•	N/A	N/A
Slovakia	1	2	2	••	•	•••	Yes
Slovenia	2	3	3	•	••	••	Yes
Spain	3	2	1	••	•	•••	No
Sweden	2	3	2	••	••	••	No
Switzerland	1	1	2	••	••	••	Yes

[a] • no education, •• short training by employer, ••• training longer than one month; [b] • 4 months or less, •• > 4 months, ••• >6 months; [c] • 2 years or less, •• between 2 and 3 years, ••• > 3 years; N/A: no information available.

Box 4.1 *Innovative ways of dealing with human resource shortages*

Several innovative practices for dealing with the shortage of human resources were mentioned by our experts.

In Bulgaria, the municipality of Sofia set up its own social assistance system as a reaction to a shortage in social assistants available through the national system. Unlike the national social assistance/home-care programmes at that time, the Sofia programme imposes hardly any requirements for the assistants (i.e. they did not have to be unemployed, they are contracted for a flexible number of hours and there may be several providers per client). Part-time work is thus possible.

The PreQual project (in Austria, the Czech Republic, Germany, Hungary and Italy) aims to fill a gap in the international education system for nursing and social-care occupations by educating migrant women to qualify them for work in the care sector. This scheme focused on the increasing need for certified nursing staff throughout Europe, and the necessity to facilitate migrant women's access to the qualified labour market, and tried to match the needs of the labour market with those of migrant women and to provide a future-oriented and innovative solution (Araujo et al., 2009).

In Slovenia, the Slovenian Federation of Pensioners Organizations developed a programme of voluntary work carried out by elderly people in order to improve their own quality of life and that of their peers. The programme involves female volunteer members of local organizations who, in their own local community, visit pensioners of 69 years and older who live at home. Having discussed with them their needs in everyday life, and if the pensioner requests assistance, the programme coordinator organizes this by informing relevant institutions (social work centre, home-care service, help at home service, Caritas or the Red Cross) of these needs. Volunteers check the implementation of assistance during a follow-up visit. Feeling lonely is often the most common problem among elderly people, so programme volunteers also help by making periodic home visits; providing various forms of nonprofessional help; or by including lonely individuals in the activities of local pensioners' organizations (Republic of Slovenia, 2008).

Telecare projects have been set up in the Netherlands. Video networks enable home-care clients and home-care providers to contact each other by use of a camera and a screen. A home-care provider can be contacted at any time, day or night. This was expected to heighten clients' sense of safety and independence and intended to substitute in part for home visits by home-care providers.

Finally, an interesting innovation that may prevent unmet needs in a context of a declining care workforce involves police officers checking on elderly people in the Czech Republic. In 'Emergency Action', an elderly person signs a contract with a police officer who takes a spare key to their house in order to ensure their well-being.

have a coordinating role). Availability of data on the actual salaries of home-care workers was fragmented, so no comprehensive overview could be drawn on this subject.

Overall, the data show that working conditions differ strongly between countries and professionals and that, generally, working conditions for domestic assistants, tend to be unfavourable – salaries tend to be low (e.g. about the minimum wage in Bulgaria, Hungary, Latvia and Portugal) and national or regional task descriptions are not available.

Unfavourable working conditions (low wages, poor fringe benefits, generally high workloads)[11] and migration are said to cause a shortage of well qualified home-care workers. For instance, home-care staff in Greece did not receive their salaries for a few months during the economic crisis of 2009/2010 and there are still insecure employment contracts.

4.5 Telecare

Telecare is an up-and-coming service across Europe (as in England, Luxembourg, the Netherlands, Portugal, Spain and Sweden). The use of telecare could result in a reduction of the human resources needed in home care or could prevent/delay admission to long-term care institutions. The use of alarm systems is fairly common in Europe – some form of alarm system is provided in about two thirds of the countries in our study. This may vary from a simple system that enables clients to press an alarm button in the case of a fall, to fairly extensive systems that use sensors to detect when a client gets out of bed or leaves the home (including GPS tracking). The use of such more advanced systems was mentioned in England, Ireland and Luxembourg. Client payments for these services are fairly common and either co-payments or fully out-of-pocket payments are required in at least 14 of the 20 countries. A second type of telecare is the video communication system which allows the client and the care provider to see each other through either a television screen or the Internet (see Box 4.1). This type of communication is mainly in the pilot phase but pilots are mentioned in Austria, Finland, the Netherlands, Norway, Slovakia and Sweden. Thus, the possibilities provided by modern communication methods seem not yet to have penetrated into home care in Europe.

4.6 Quality monitoring, management and improvement

Quality monitoring and quality management have become common (although not universal) practices in health systems in Europe. But this is not always the

---

11 Austria, Belgium, Czech Republic, France, Greece, Lithuania and Slovenia.

case in home care, especially in those parts of home care that might be regarded as non-personal support, such as domestic aid. This section explores the range of approaches used by countries to monitor (and possibly improve) home care, using data from three key areas – (i) whether, and how, countries use quality measures to assess care provision, at either organizational or individual level; (ii) how monitoring of quality assessment is carried out; and (iii) whether and how client or carer complaints and concerns are used to improve service provision.

There are clear links between the organization of quality assessment at different levels and governance. Both deal with issues such as accreditation of agencies, certification of providers and user choice. However, because this analysis is focused rather on the framework of systems and tools for quality improvement, only brief mention will be made of the uses to which the quality measurement results may be put. In Chapter 2, the regulation of quality of care is addressed in the context of accreditation requirements, certification of providers and user choice. In this section, we further elaborate on the subject at the level of the organization of care.

4.6.1 Quality measures and measurement

Where quality measures do exist, they are often in the form of quality standards (e.g. the expected standard of personal care to be provided). Explicitly stated quality standards are increasingly being proposed as the basis for assessing the structure of services (are they fit for purpose?); the quality (with security issues embedded) and effectiveness of the care process; and the impact (outcome) of care services. But there are a number of caveats. The methodology of assessing quality is still evolving, so measures are often developed for the organizational, rather than the personal, level of care. Also, these measures still tend to be about structure and process of care, rather than outcome. Individual-based tools do exist – such as the resident assessment instrument (RAI) (interRAI, 2007) and the Barthel index – but few countries report the use of these instruments. The RAI is used in some Nordic countries for determining change over time for people who live in residential accommodation, but these have been rarely used (or at least reported on) in the home-care sector (only in Austria, Iceland, Norway and Switzerland). In parts of Austria, the use of the Residents Assessment Instrument for Home Care (RAI HC) is mandatory. The use of the Barthel index is reported in Spain and Lithuania and in a modified form in Poland. In Portugal, the quality management system of the European Foundation for Quality Management is the preferred model for social home care, but its use is not obligatory. Uniform monitoring procedures facilitate the assessment of provision, outcomes and effectiveness, and comparability among not only providers but also countries.

At a national level, Denmark and several other countries are developing explicit criteria. Although still at the pilot or feasibility stage, the Danish standards are based on national guidelines for home-care services (including personal care and domestic care), using 23 indicators for assessments. The outcome indicators are based partly on yearly surveys among receivers of home care (e.g. perception of quality and continuity of care); the process indicators are based on activities, content and expenses. Additionally – under an established system in Sweden – indicators for good care, and quality assessed at the municipality level, are subjected to national comparison in the expectation that this will improve overall quality. Similarly, the Netherlands has Quality Norms for Home Care. In Belgium, Finland and France more general standards are laid down in a quality framework. England also used an extensive set of social home-care indicators allied to inspection (excluding domestic care) until 2010 but these have been withdrawn as a result of national policy changes. Self-assessment by the provider has since been the main regulatory process, although recent concerns about quality of care and poor regulation will lead to the reinstatement of provider inspections. The Spanish national system also uses process and outcome indicators for the home health services, but not for the domestic aid component of home care. In France, the new accreditation agency (Agence nationale de l'évaluation et de la qualité des établissements et services sociaux et médico-sociaux – ANESM) is developing a set of indicators for this latter area.

More commonly, where national home-care standards exist (as in the Polish national system) they are targeted at structural issues such as requirements for staff qualifications, standard equipment and standards of premises. These standards are often minimum rather than optimal. Thus, for example, until recently the Irish health and social home-care system has only collected data on the number of state-funded staffing hours provided for professional and domestic care and has had no quality review system in place for home care.

Measures to increase the quality of domestic aid seem to exist only rarely, perhaps due to the very wide range of provision. These services are often purchased locally or are provided mainly by families, as is the case in countries as widely dispersed as Spain, Austria, Italy and Bulgaria. Among other things, this situation of limited quality assessment also occurs because it is more difficult for regulators to scrutinize the quality of care provision when carers are hired and employed directly by the family. This situation is likely to extend with the introduction of personal care budgets (e.g. as reported in Greece).

4.6.2 Quality assessment

Most European countries have some form of quality assessment for home care enshrined in legislation or regulation. These rules are usually targeted at provider organizations, whether directly state funded or commissioned through some other means. Many of these quality systems are at 'arms-length' through commissioning. Providers are funded only when they agree to meet a level of standards or authorization (see also Section 2.2). These systems may be quite complicated. For instance, three types of home-care agency assessment exist in France: (i) 'authorization' delivered by the executive body of the local political level (*conseil général*); (ii) 'agreement' delivered by the state local representative (*préfet*); and (iii) 'certification' delivered by the national care agency (ANESM).

A few countries have national semi-independent assessment authorities, such as the Care Quality Commission (CQC) in England, which until 2010 undertook both registration and inspections of providers. In Norway, the Norwegian Board of Health Supervision continuously assesses whether institutions, home-care districts or other services have good quality systems for providing health care. In the Netherlands, the Health Care Inspectorate (IGZ) is responsible for the supervision of the quality of services. Home-care agencies are legally obliged to systematically monitor and improve the quality of their services and staff and to provide annual reports to the IGZ. An audit is performed when the IGZ expects quality problems based on these reports; the IGZ does not act proactively. In contrast, health inspectors from the Danish regional health authorities pay unannounced visits once per year, inspecting local guidelines and other documents as well as interviewing residents and health personnel.

There are a number of challenges in establishing quality assessment systems in home care. For some countries the priority is considered greater in the health-care sector, with personal care and domestic aid either falling on informal caregivers or home-care service quality management being given a low priority. Furthermore, since many home health and social home-care systems are in transition, the quality assessment processes also may be subject to change. Ireland is now developing criteria for assessing the quality of providers for home-care services provided by the state. At the same time, there is the challenge of how to regulate the quality of home-care providers coming from the private sector. Regionalization may produce some problems in this regard. Hence, in France, quality assessment is not always undertaken on a similar basis at the local (*conseil général*) level even if standards are national. Changing political priorities in England mean that quality assessment visits by the CQC were stopped; evidence in the following period of redesign showed widespread quality concerns. Germany has mandated highly controversial public reporting on the quality of long-term care facilities and home-care agencies (care grades

– *Pflegenoten*) as a result of the quality assessment carried out by the medical service of the health-care funds at least once a year.

Where a country has political federalization (e.g. as in Austria, Belgium or Switzerland), any quality assessment system tends to be specific to the individual states. An exception is reported in Germany, where the quality assessment is carried out by a semi-independent institution using criteria applying to the whole nation. The same phenomenon may occur when responsibilities have been delegated to municipalities, which may result in variations within the country. This may also mean that national frameworks for the implementation of quality systems (established at a policy level) do not furnish the expected information on the quality of care. Italy faces such a challenge where audits of the service (when made) are executed by the social services of the municipality and by the regional health service managers of integrated health services (ADI) involved in the home.

Quality assessment at the individual level is written into regulations in different ways. Many countries have professional regulatory systems for client security that apply to both home health care and social home care. These relate particularly to incidents relating to the professional work of nurses and doctors and also apply to the work of professionals in home care. For example, in Denmark and France it is now mandatory for personnel to report unforeseen events in all areas of home care; in Sweden it is mandatory for personnel to report neglect and mismanagement of older people. It is unusual for quality assessment to be undertaken by individual staff; they only check whether care is consistent with the client care plan. For example, although the health component seems to be given a higher priority than the social/domestic component of care in most systems, individual clinical staff such as nurses and therapists do not undertake local quality assessments (as distinct from case management evaluation); where local quality audits occur they are carried out by dedicated or more senior staff. However, in a few states the assessment of quality seems more significant in the social home-care sector than in the health sector. For instance, Latvia has a layered system of quality review from state level to the use of municipal quality specialists who visit clients once a year; the quality of nursing care relies mainly on informal review by the client's GP.

Evidence gathered during the study suggests that there may be significant differences between developing a quality assessment system and its implementation. The most obvious examples of variable implementation seem to arise when the process is devolved to a regional or municipal level, or when multiple providers are commissioned and a quality assessment system is required of them – but not always carried out. One, though by no means the only, example of variation at regional level can be drawn from Italy, where the quality of services varies considerably among local health authorities and municipalities, and there is a lack of common tools for client evaluation and quality monitoring. Explicit monitoring procedures of delivered services (e.g. to address the worsening of a clinical situation) are uncommon.

Overall, a picture appears of some excellent and comprehensive practices across the whole of home care and of some good practice in assessing the quality of home-care nursing. However, there seems to be considerable variation in extent. Furthermore, reorganization and policy changes continue to result in gaps and uncertainties in quality assessment. And while many countries have arrangements for assessing the quality of the 'health' component of home care (e.g. for personal care for people with complex needs or nursing or rehabilitation care), there is much less focus on the quality of domestic care.

4.6.3 Home-care professionals involved in quality assessments

Home-care professionals or organizations are often involved in the monitoring of the actual provision of care and reassessment of care needs. In around one third of the countries,[12] this reassessment of needs is delegated to special officers or organizations who may be commissioned by the municipality (as in Denmark and Finland); may be health-care workers, such as a GP, qualified nurse or primary care team (as in England, Hungary, Ireland and Slovakia); or may be social workers (England and Ireland).

The frequency of reassessment varies widely between the countries. In Hungary, needs are reassessed after 14 visits of the home nurse; in Latvia, reassessment occurs every month (although there is no formal regulation requiring this). In Slovenia, reassessments occur every three months; England and Finland maintain a six-month period; and Austria, France and Sweden reassess yearly. In the Netherlands, reassessment of some cases may occur after five years. Half of the countries report that the carer can report changing needs between assessments and that this can lead to a change in the care provided.

A similar picture can be drawn for social home care. In just over one third of the countries,[13] special officers or organizations (often connected with municipalities or national governments) monitor care and provide reassessments of care needs. In Belgium (Flanders), England, Estonia, France and the Netherlands, providers also make self-assessments of the quality of care.

---

12 Austria, Czech Republic, Denmark, England, Finland, Germany, Greece, Hungary, Romania, Slovakia and Slovenia.

13 Austria, Bulgaria, Cyprus, Czech Republic, England, Finland, Germany, Iceland, Malta, Poland, Romania, Slovakia and Sweden.

4.6.4 Quality improvement through client involvement

Two other types of contribution to quality improvement are increasingly being taken into account – complaints and solicited comments on satisfaction with services (see also Chapter 3).

Most, but not all (see following paragraphs), countries have incorporated client-centred complaints processes into their home-care services. When services are provided by, or are under the direct control of, the state there is usually a very formal system. This system may be similar to that used for other parts of the health service, with a process of escalation from local conciliation to a regional or even state level of response. Where services are commissioned by the state or other agencies, providers are required to have a complaints service in place although the commissioner usually has little or no actual involvement.

Information on the means of complaint may sometimes be hard to access for both clients and family carers. Sometimes the state, but more frequently charities and the non-profit-making sector, assist with the provision of advice and support with the complaints procedure.

For home health care, formal complaints procedures exist in almost all countries in our study. Only two countries reported explicitly that no such possibility was available (Greece and Iceland). In about one third of the countries,[14] complaints procedures are the responsibility of the care provider. In the Netherlands, the care provider is expected to install an independent complaints commission; in Portugal, providers are required to provide a book of complaints that clients may read upon request. In the Scandinavian countries, complaints should be filed with the municipality or the regional or national government (in Finland, Norway and Sweden). In about one third of the countries studied,[15] special regional or national institutes are in place for handling clients' complaints. For instance, one possibility in the Netherlands is to file complaints against individual care providers through the disciplinary boards set up by the professions. Other examples can be found in the country reports.

Social home care shows similar variations in complaints procedures as home nursing care. However, more countries mentioned that there are no formal complaints procedures (Austria, Croatia, Greece, Ireland and Lithuania). Furthermore, fewer countries have regional or national institutes involved in handling complaints. Options to appeal in cases where the (mostly provider-based) complaints procedure does not settle the complaint satisfactorily were reported in the Czech Republic, Lithuania, Luxembourg, the Netherlands, Norway and Romania.

---

14 Belgium (Flanders), Czech Republic, England, Estonia, Germany, Italy, Luxembourg, the Netherlands, Portugal, Slovakia, Spain and Switzerland.

15 Belgium (Flanders, for complaints on the assignment of care), Bulgaria, Croatia, Cyprus, Latvia, Lithuania, Luxembourg, the Netherlands, Poland and Slovakia.

Evaluation of client satisfaction as a component of service quality evaluation seems to be expanding, although perhaps more slowly than the establishment of complaints processes. The structural use of client surveys was reported in Belgium (Flanders), Finland, France, the Netherlands, Norway, Portugal and Slovenia. These surveys are not always mandatory (as in Portugal) nor implemented nationwide (as in Latvia and Slovenia). Incidental satisfaction surveys were carried out in Belgium, Cyprus, Denmark, England, Ireland and Luxembourg.

For EU countries, the Special Eurobarometer (2007) interviews with clients and carers can provide an interesting comparative overview of satisfaction with services although the individual country sample sizes are not large and there are no data on intra-country variation (TNS Opinion and Social, 2007). Some smaller states seem to undertake few, or only occasional, studies of satisfaction, or are only beginning to explore these issues in other parts of the primary care system (e.g. in Ireland). In general, no client satisfaction surveys of social home care are reported in Estonia, Greece and Spain. The use of client surveys varies among the autonomous communities in Spain but generally is poor. However, home health services have satisfaction surveys related to all primary care services, including home care.

Notwithstanding the above, there are considerable doubts over the extent to which the results of the whole 'satisfaction survey industry' are used to monitor or improve services.

4.6.5 Models of quality management

A considerable range of quality system processes can be found in quality management in the 31 study countries and there is often an overlap between different parts of the systems found in different areas of quality management between different countries. Yet it is possible to discern some contrasting generic models which can be categorized as a centralized model, a regulatory model and a distributed model (see Table 4.6). These models should be interpreted as ideal types as, in practice, there will be overlaps between the models within countries – for example, where a regulatory model lacks control and effectively becomes a distributed model.

4.7 Challenges and developments

4.7.1 Developments in home-care delivery

In several north-western European countries,[16] budget shortages are causing

---

16 France, Iceland, the Netherlands, Scandinavian countries and Switzerland.

Table 4.6 *Three broad models of quality management*

Centralized	Regulatory	Distributed
Features		
Dominant role of national government	State or national care system funded agency or agencies	Weak regulatory role of national government or state/system-wide agencies
National vision or laws	Strong regulatory role	No, or limited, national regulatory framework
Detailed requirements and processes set by national governments	Agencies act within a framework of national laws or regulations	Limited protections for service users
State imposes sanctions or restrictions for poor provider performance	Agencies apply common regulatory standards across the nation/state	Responsibilities, regulation and practices devolved, or left to, regions, municipalities or communities
	Agencies have regulatory powers to impose sanctions or restrictions for poor provider performance or serious complaints	Sector-initiated regional or national standards
		Quality control and assessment first responsibility of providers
Actors		
Central government sets detailed regulation and/or laws	Provider self-regulation with national reporting and agency overview	Providers, both state and private, setting their own rules or working under 'light touch' regulation
National inspection services, possibly devolved, but reporting upwards	Professional bodies or provider associations taking responsibility for some aspects of quality and performance review	Limited or no feedback at state level and little or no public reporting of results by providers
National quality systems may publish results of inspections or data on quality issues	Possibly more control of state-managed providers than of private providers	Inspection agencies come into play when assessments show poor results

governments to ration services. At the same time, certain services are being extended or are planned to be extended in 19 countries. Mostly, these increases relate to the provision of home nursing[17] or to home care in general. In several countries the increase pertains mainly to specialized services, such as palliative care at home.[18]

Linked to governments' rationing of services, growth in the private provision sector is a widespread development. However, this change is far from uniform across countries. Existing private provision is expanding[19] and new providers are entering the market. In some southern European countries, the expansion of private provision is supported mainly by an increase in the number of migrant

---
17 As in Bulgaria, Cyprus, Estonia, Hungary, Ireland, Latvia, Lithuania and Poland.

18 As in the Netherlands and Norway and specifically for palliative care in, for example, Belgium, France, Lithuania, Luxembourg, Poland, Portugal, Slovenia and Spain.

19 For example, NGOs in Cyprus and Bulgaria.

workers from other countries (e.g. in the social care systems of Cyprus, Greece, Italy and Malta). These workers are mostly untrained, may be illegal and may have language problems. In the Scandinavian countries, home care was previously provided only by public providers but private organizations (both profit-making and non-profit-making) are entering the market. Sometimes this is encouraged as a matter of national policy and seems to be for diverse reasons, such as to complement the shortage of public provision or to encourage more efficient behaviour of public providers. Another important reason seems to be to ration publicly funded domestic aid services. In Finland and Sweden, for instance, some basic domestic aid is publicly funded. Those needing or wanting more turn to the private sector. In Belgium, the growing private provision pertains to the social home-care sector; in Ireland it relates to both the personal care and domestic aid sectors. In some countries it was suggested that one reason for the public sector's proportionate decrease in the market was that it was more profitable for professionals to work independently or in the private sector (e.g. in Belgium and the Czech Republic).

Another major and important development regarding the care process is governments' efforts to increase their control over the quality of home care. This has been done partly because of the low quality of services perceived by clients, sometimes related to safety of care issues. In about half of the countries studied this seemed a current policy issue. For example, either there have been plans to increase educational requirements for home-care professionals or such requirements were introduced recently (as in Bulgaria and Cyprus); new quality control mechanisms have been introduced (in Estonia and Portugal); quality certificates for care providers have been developed (in Austria); and special official national quality frameworks have come into effect (in Belgium, Finland Luxembourg and the Netherlands). These frameworks lay down the concept of quality and some quality norms, but generally these norms remain vaguely described.

Quality management is an area closely linked to all of the other themes in this report. Possibly that makes quality management one of the high priorities for collaboration and improvement across the whole community of European countries.

While it is clear that there is a move towards assessing the quality of home-care services in many European countries, there are significant implementation difficulties. Those countries that are still building their health and social care provision from a low base have limited quality systems in place for home care and seem to give these services low priority. There are also some larger or more affluent countries where implementation varies or is at an early stage. Reporting on the quality of home care happens in only a few countries. These countries have national, transparent schemes and publish results on the Internet. Satisfaction surveys exist in some countries, but are used by providers only for internal use. On the whole, reporting on quality and client satisfaction is an area that needs attention and improvement in Europe.

Whether taken by providers themselves or by governments, initiatives to increase coordination between home-care services, and between home care and other types of health care, take the form of introducing multidisciplinary care teams; formal cooperation between providers or services, case managers, shared care plans and information systems; and coordinated care pathways. Additionally, in a few countries, efforts are being made to lay down clear regulator, funder and provider responsibilities. In most countries, however, coordination is not built into the structure of the home-care organization and/or is left to the initiative of providers. Therefore, this is another area that needs attention and improvement in Europe.

The use of basic telecare may also increase the possibilities of remaining at home, although the use of this type of care is still in its infancy in Europe. There are several pilots in different countries but little evidence of the regular use of telecare is reported in the literature so far. Nevertheless, our experts identified some countries in which there is already extensive use of the new technologies which are cheap and easy to install.

4.7.2 Current concerns

The anticipated shortage of (qualified) home-care professionals seems to be a significant problem. In parallel with financial shortages, limited supplies of trained staff are seen as the cause of unmet needs in many countries in Europe. A general shortage of home-care staff existed in several countries[20] as well as a lack of (sufficiently qualified) home-care staff.[21] Unfavourable working conditions – such as low wages, poor fringe benefits or generally high workloads[22] – and migration of people from low-wage countries to higher-wage countries, are two of the main causes.

Europe faces a challenge in trying to increase manpower for home-care services. To increase human resources quickly, some countries may initially have to lower their educational standards and this may jeopardize the quality of care. A lack of personnel resulted in the use of more unskilled labour in Denmark. In Luxembourg, the expansion of the home-care sector has also resulted in personnel being hired with a lower level of qualification. Hence, investments in the professionalization of home-care staff (i.e. training, adequate qualification,

---

20 Austria, Belgium, Bulgaria, Cyprus, Czech Republic, Finland, France, Greece, Lithuania, Portugal and Slovenia.
21 Bulgaria, Cyprus, Denmark, Estonia, France, Germany, Greece, Luxembourg and Norway.
22 Austria, Belgium, Czech Republic, France, Greece, Lithuania and Slovenia.

new models of qualification and development of ethical standards) and safeguarding of conditions of employment need to be considered. Additionally, as informal care is increasingly important and being professionalized, the introduction of training and social security may also be a relevant policy option for this group. Foreign (migrant) workers may offer a partial solution to the manpower problem but they often lack appropriate educational qualifications. Thus, investment in the education of this group is necessary if they are to contribute to improved staffing levels.

Task substitution was mentioned in some countries as an important development. For example, in Denmark, tasks formerly in the hands of GPs are now in the hands of nurses; and tasks formerly in the hands of nurses are now the duty of nursing assistants. In the Netherlands, a similar substitution is also taking place in domestic aid. The question arising in the countries with widespread task substitution is whether, and how, this affects the quality of care.

In some countries the lack of (private) agencies was mentioned as problematic. The home-care sector was seen as unattractive for new providers – for instance, due to reimbursement levels that are considered to be unviable. Little is known about the client-financed home-care sector (extent of need, size of the sector, types of organization involved and extent and quality of the care provided), but it seems to be growing in several countries. Further work is required to try to understand how this market is emerging.

The decreasing availability of residential care services leads to higher pressure on available home-care services, and is happening relatively fast in some countries.[23] For example, where more restrictive eligibility criteria are introduced for residential care, there needs to be a concomitant increase for relevant, possibly higher level, home-care provision. If not, care provision for clients who need more intensive levels of care may become problematic.

In many countries, concerns were raised about the lack of integration between home health care and home social care. Generally, this lack of integration in the delivery of health and social services is also associated with a lack of integration in the needs assessment and monitoring of the quality of services. In almost all countries it is common practice that different types of home care are provided by different organizations or teams. Often, home-care coordination takes place voluntarily and this, by its very nature, puts services at risk. As we have shown, formal coordination between home care and hospital care is stronger than coordination between home care and nursing home/residential care. In some places there are weak links between home health care and home social care.

---

23 For example, Finland, Iceland, Ireland and Poland.

However, there are good examples of integrated care across Europe and these can be drawn on as possible models for developing systems.

As already discussed, the need to ensure good quality of care is a widespread European issue.[24] There are concerns that the quality of care may be endangered by the lack of time available for professionals/providers to provide the necessary care at home. Many efforts are being made across Europe to tackle these problems. However, in some countries, country experts currently have some concerns about the lack of grip on the quality of care. Nationwide or internationally comparative data often are not available. Furthermore, the use of client surveys is increasing but not yet common practice; where these are in place, it does not automatically lead to freely available publication of the results. Complaints procedures are often in place but it is not clear whether these function satisfactorily in practice.

Concerns were also raised about the poor conditions for enabling older people or people with disabilities to continue to live in their own homes. Adequate adapted housing was said to be scarce in several countries; availability of day-care places and respite care was variable in others. It is common to find that home adaptations also are not fully publically financed.

4.8 Overview and policy issues

Management policy and practice for the home-care sector is in transition in many countries. This chapter has identified key areas on which policy-makers and home-care managers may focus. Investing in the profession of home-care workers or in formalizing informal care may be considered. Furthermore, continued efforts are needed across Europe to ensure a situation in which the provision of a range of adapted housing enables as many people as possible to remain living in the community.

Efforts are needed to reduce unmet needs (both health and social needs) and care discontinuity. Home-care managers and policy-makers could invest further in exploring and solving problems in care continuity and inefficient overlaps; and generally in integrating social and health sectors at all levels, in both care provision and governance. Furthermore, in many countries, 'quality' remains undefined or defined only vaguely. As long as there is no common understanding of quality – and hence no common quality norms – it will be difficult for governments to control quality, especially given the growing number of private providers.

---

24 Belgium, Bulgaria, Croatia, France, Germany, Hungary, Iceland, Italy, Latvia, the Netherlands, Portugal, Romania, Slovakia, Slovenia, Spain and Switzerland.

Private providers often add to the basic services provided by publicly owned or financed home care. The share of private provision is increasing in Europe. Private providers are interested in providing home-care services in some countries but have no interest in entering into home-care provision in countries with unfavourable market conditions. In these countries there may be a risk of unmet needs (in addition to other risks of unmet needs, such as affordability problems). Nevertheless, competition that has regulatory oversight may offer wider choice to clients and has been shown to extend the range of care on offer. There may be models here that could offer a basis for development within home-care systems in transition.

The nature of the private sector providing care directly to clients (i.e. those without the support of formal needs assessments or public funding) is often unknown to policy-makers. These private providers may also operate outside of a regulatory framework or may be privately hired but paid through public funds in the form of personal budgets. Development of an effective and efficient home-care sector requires a better understanding of the interrelationship between private providers contracted directly by clients and more formalized services.

Last, but no means least, there is the pressing issue of an adequate supply of trained and valued home-care professionals. This is perhaps the highest priority at a European level among all of the other issues raised in this chapter on the management of the home-care sector.

References

Afrite A et al. (2007). Hospital at home, an economical alternative for rehabilitative care. *Questions d'économie de la santé*, 119:1–8.

Araujo T et al. (2009). *PreQual basics. International prequalification for migrant women entering into the health and care sector*. Linz, Maiz (http://prequalsteps.maiz.at/en/system/files/PreQual_basics_EN.pdf, accessed 5 June 2012).

Grilz-Wolf M et al. (2004). Providing integrated health and social care for older persons in Austria. In: Alaszewski A, Leichsenring K, eds. *Providing integrated health and social care for older persons: a European overview of issues at stake*. Aldershot, Ashgate Publishing:97–138.

interRAI (2007). *interRAI HC – Home Care*. Ann Arbor, interRAI (http://www.interrai.org/ index.php?id=94, accessed 28 August 2012).

Republic of Slovenia (2008). *National report on strategies for social protection and social inclusion 2008–2010*. Ljubljana, Republic of Slovenia:46

TNS Opinion & Social (2007). Health and long-term care in the European Union. Brussels, European Commission, *Special Eurobarometer 283/Wave 67.3*.

Chapter 5
Conclusions and the way forward

Nadine Genet, Wienke Boerma, Madelon Kroneman, Allen Hutchinson

Substantial inter-country variations in available services and diversity in the organization of home nursing, personal care and domestic aid provided in clients' home were evident throughout the previous chapters. At the same time we have seen similarities in the tough challenges for the home-care sector across Europe that demand action from decision-makers. This chapter will focus on these challenges, which may also turn out to be opportunities, and discuss ways in which the sector may move forward.

5.1 Complexity of the home-care sector

The picture of home care as it emerged from the literature – a complex sector with a large variation in governance, financing and delivery – has been confirmed and detailed by the findings of this study. We found a wide range of services provided in patients' homes, including long-term care, short-term recuperation after hospital discharge and palliative care, and both social and health-care services. Governance structures and organization were fragmented and borders between types of services were sometimes blurred.

Fragmentation on the one hand, and strong links and interdependency between home care and various other sectors on the other, mean that decisions or policy shifts regarding home care may have indirect and sometimes unexpected effects in neighbouring sectors such as hospitals, nursing homes and social work. The fragmented character of home care is the reason why it is more justified to speak about it as a sector rather than a system. It consists of subsectors characterized as professional and reimbursed or volunteer and unpaid; profit-making or non-profit-making; publicly owned and publicly regulated or privately regulated. Such differences strongly influence the possibilities for governments to steer the sector. The hybrid private sector may be hard to control as it may consist of non-profit-making (usually charitable) organizations financed by a mix of gifts and public and private resources; private profit-making organizations financed by public and/or private resources; or completely privately financed and profit-making providers. It may be easier to steer private providers if they are contracted to the publicly financed home-care system.

5.1.1 Governance

Although most countries have developed a vision on home care at national level, such national visions are neither detailed nor homogenous and governance and decision-making are typically strongly decentralized. Lack of homogeneity relates partly to the different roots of home health care (nursing) and social home care (domestic aid) – usually, visions have been developed separately for these two pillars of home care. More detailed visions are found with local governments. What have been laid down at a national level are principles, general entitlements and possible restrictions. For instance, entitlements to home care for people with insufficient means and for other vulnerable groups are often set nationally. Restrictions may be concerned with price limits and defining groups who need to receive home care free of charge. Principles may state the importance of quality and the need to assure the quality and responsiveness of services. Within these frameworks set at national level, local governments or private organizations are left to design and implement details.

5.1.2 Financing

European countries spent on average 0.6% of their health-care expenditures on curative home and rehabilitative home care and 3.5% on long-term nursing care at home (Eurostat, 08-12-2010). Figures on home care within the social-care system (mostly domestic aid) are rarely available and statistics on private home-care expenditure are absent in many countries, especially those types of care paid out-of-pocket by clients.

There is a wide variation in how financing is organized within countries. Different types of home care are financed differently and from several different sources. The two main methods of home-care funding are either: (i) a combination of taxation for home social care and health insurance for home nursing care; or (ii) a combination of taxation for home nursing care and social insurance for home social care. Only two countries (Germany, the Netherlands) have specific long-term care insurance in place.

Means tested client co-payments are usual in most countries. Means testing can aim either to collect higher contributions from those with higher incomes or to provide (publicly funded) care free of charge to those with lower incomes. This may result in fully out-of-pocket payments for those above a certain income ceiling.

5.1.3 Clients in focus

Although all European countries have some home-care infrastructure and provide publicly funded home-care services to some extent, various unmet needs could be identified. Some types of services can be underrepresented in countries or regions within countries – for instance, psychological support and psychosocial care. Also, certain population groups may be underserved due to financial restraint, prevailing eligibility criteria or differences in the availability of informal carers. Deficits in formal care are usually compensated for by informal caregivers. However, the division of tasks between the formal and informal systems depends on cultural values; the composition of families; and attitudes concerning ageing and the place of older people in society (e.g. the importance of staying independent). Information on unmet needs is rarely available.

At present, especially in southern countries, people who consider themselves to be in need of care prefer informal care. But, even in countries where the preference is more towards professional care, informal carers are and will continue to be essential in home care. Safeguarding the potential of informal caregivers will thus become a major challenge for future governments. This will be a central issue – whether being an informal caregiver is a real choice or a position more or less forced on carers by a lack of alternatives. Finding an optimal balance between informal and formal carers will be another challenge. Organized support and relief for informal caregivers was not available in most countries.

5.1.4 The management perspective

Generally, many *types* of home-care services are available but often not very extensively. Clients generally would be able to access relatively extensive services in Austria, Belgium, Denmark, England, Ireland, Luxembourg, the Netherlands, Norway and Sweden. The other countries have considerable needs that remain unaddressed by formally provided services.

Although the main type of home-care provider is still public, private providers of home care are available in almost all countries and their involvement seems to be increasing in several countries. A wide range of providers is working in the privately financed home-care sector. The two main groups within this sector are NGOs and other similar organizations (relying on gifts or public funding) and completely privately financed services (through private insurance or out-of-pocket payments). Most of the information available on private providers relates to those services with the support of public money.

In most countries different types of agency are involved in the provision of home care, each usually providing only part of the palette of services (e.g. only domestic assistance or home nursing). Formal coordination of services is unusual. Generally, coordination of home-care services is voluntary and *incidental*. Coordination with home care is strongest for the transition from hospital care to home care and still rather weak at the interface with nursing homes. It is important to distinguish between home help and home nursing, as coordination between nursing care and other health-care providers is usually better than that between home help and other health-care providers. In general, formal integration of home care with other health-care provision is most developed in England, Italy, the Netherlands, Scandinavian countries and Slovakia, and least formally integrated in Bulgaria, France and Romania.

Quality monitoring and quality management are not routine in home care, especially regarding non-personal support such as domestic aid.

5.2 Taking on the challenge

A major concern in the home-care sector across Europe relates to the challenge of how to cope with growing demand in a time of financial constraints and shortages of professional human resources. Most EU countries seem to be fighting a losing battle in trying to meet fully the demand for home care with the current capacity. In many cases, de-institutionalization policies have compounded the negative influences of a lack of funding and unfavourable working conditions, especially for domestic aides. For the countries in central and eastern Europe, the current period of shrinking public resources is further delaying the development of early home-care systems. The key to solutions may be found in a combination of innovation and a fundamental improvement of efficiency.

Balancing quality, costs and lack of human resources

Shortages of human resources in the home-care sector are foreseen in all countries but only a few seem to have prepared. Where this preparation has occurred, a range of different strategies has been developed. Some countries have responded to shortages of home-care workers by lowering the educational requirements (e.g. Luxembourg and Austria) or by offering on-the-job training (as in Latvia). Another approach is delegation of tasks from higher to lower educated (and cheaper) home-care workers. For instance, task substitution from physicians to nurses and from nurses to home help has been tried. Possible pitfalls of delegation and substitution include compromises on the quality of care. Particularly in countries where educational requirements and standards for social-care functions are not well developed or not well maintained, a lack of qualified home-care staff has already been reported. Task substitution can be a remedy on a limited scale but its longer-term viability may be questioned as increased costs for coordination, supervision and training may threaten initial efficiency gains.

Governments will face the dilemma of balancing the short-term need for human resources with the need to maintain professional standards. Probably more promising are attempts to enhance flexibility, improve the integration of different types of services and develop effective structures to support informal care and self-care. The application of new technology in these approaches would require additional initial investments but eventually could contribute to solving the human resources problem.

5.2.1 Targeting financial resources

In order to further curb the state costs of home care, countries have introduced additional financial contributions and tightened up eligibility criteria. Irrespective of the mode of home-care funding (taxation, social insurance or a mix of both), some out-of-pocket payment is required in most countries to prevent overuse and control cost. These cost containment measures create new obstacles to the utilization of home care which may particularly affect vulnerable groups and thus threaten equity. Means testing is common in a number of countries, either pertaining to the level of client co-payments or to controlling access to publicly funded services. In the latter case, certain groups may not be able to use services if market prices are high. Additionally, there may be quality differences between services provided by the privately financed sector and those from the publicly financed sector. Besides, solidarity may be at stake where governments reduce the eligibility for publicly funded services more and more. If relatively few people benefit from publicly funded services then public support may erode and, consequently, the willingness to pay for services may decrease. To prevent inequity in access and quality, standards of service quality or maximum prices can be imposed on private providers. However, such measures include costs for developing regulations and monitoring adherence and bear the risk of overregulation.

Although governments in some countries have extended the range of publicly funded home-care services (e.g. by offering palliative care at home as a substitute for hospital care) the trend is towards rationing, especially in the western European countries. Cutting the package of home-care services is the dominant response to financial constraints. This affects both informal caregivers and those in need of care. Many partners and family members will have no choice but to contribute more, either practically or financially. Many of those in need of care will probably become more dependent on their families and – if the ability or willingness to pay or to care is lacking – the result will be that their needs for care will not be fully met.

Some countries (such as Belgium, Croatia and the Netherlands) have planned systematic identification of areas of rationing through more transparency in the allocation of funds. However, it is not certain whether the expected savings will balance the costs of transparency. For example, domestic aid may reduce the risk of falling and, indirectly, the resulting need for personal care or even nursing. But attempts to target resources more towards preventive home visits and preventive care in general could be at the expense of people with extensive immediate needs for care. In addition, some consider that decentralized decision-making may be more efficient as it tailors home care more to local needs; others consider that it may be quite inefficient as municipalities have to reinvent the wheel. Information exchange and the distribution of good ideas between municipalities may be helpful in preventing inefficiencies in such systems.

5.2.2 Geographical equity

Throughout Europe the governance of home care is largely decentralized. National governments have developed visions on home care, including purpose, minimum availability, costs and general entitlements. Such 'framework' regulations are elaborated by lower levels of government or NGOs. In many countries local authorities have considerable responsibility and discretion for designing home-care systems in their areas, particularly for social home-care services. This may result in great differences within countries as municipalities may not be prepared for these new tasks – the local level is often too small to have the necessary expertise and information. In such cases decentralization may rather increase inequity and regional differences rather than be a means to better serve local populations.

Disparities between urban and rural areas in the provision of home-care services were manifest in several countries. Rural populations are underserved with home care because of lack of transportation and less developed infrastructures. Furthermore, rural populations are ageing as younger people migrate to cities and abroad. This results in relatively high needs for care on the one hand and a lack of personnel for home care and of informal caregivers on the other. It is difficult for national policy-makers to tackle this growing imbalance but

they can set minimum requirements, monitor differences and influence local authorities.

5.2.3 Safeguarding coordination

Another typical feature of the home-care sector in almost all countries[1] is the different governance structures for the three streams of domestic aid, personal care and nursing care. This fragmented governance is a cause of poor coordination in cases that require more than one type of care. Social home care is decentralized more often than home health care. Additionally, national-level responsibility for social home care and home health care usually resides under different ministries and thus different legislation, regulations and financing schemes apply. As a consequence, the delivery of home health care and home social care may be poorly integrated. Overall, it may be concluded that coordination of home-care services is rather an exception than the rule. This could be tackled by investing in multiprofessional teamwork, an approach that has been shown to be successful.

Intersectoral coordination between home health care and hospitals is relatively well developed. Social workers and liaison nurses working in the context of protocols and agreements are important ingredients. However, such arrangements are not well developed between home care and nursing homes and there are lessons to be learned from the home care/hospital processes.

Nevertheless, in most countries, coordination between home care and other care providers – including hospitals – relates mainly to home health care rather than home social care. Positive exceptions are the Scandinavian countries where both types of services are also integrated at governance and provision levels. In addition to these countries, formal integration of home care and other health-care provision is best developed in England, the Netherlands and Slovakia.

5.2.4 'Marketing'

A cause of unmet needs in home care is the disconnection between demand and supply. Potential clients and even referring professionals may not be familiar with available home-care services. The visibility of home care may be improved by setting up a one-stop information window (either physically or on the Internet) for potential clients and carers and, at the same time, improving information to key referring providers (e.g. GPs, social workers, community nurses) or posting case managers between clients and the services.

---

1 Except Denmark, Greece, Sweden and some parts of Portugal and Finland.

As home care is largely decentralized, insight into the problems of the sector at central level is not optimal and will not be improved by the trend of increasing private home-care provision. Little is known about services provided by the privately financed sector; the quality of care; and the costs of its services, especially where care is purchased without any public intermediary. Additionally, personal budgets enable clients to purchase care, if so desired, from private or public providers and from professionals or non-professionals. The multitude of care options will make insight and, hence, quality control more complex. A comprehensive policy on home care should include a duty for governments to at least monitor services provided in the private sector and understand possible gaps between the publicly funded, regulated and privately funded subsectors. Policy-makers could consider introducing uniform reporting requirements on the care process for both the public and private sectors. Private providers may need to be more accountable for the number, type and education of professionals working in their agencies.

5.2.5 Balancing regulation, flexibility and efficiency

Currently, home care provided by private (profit-making or non-profit-making) agencies is the dominant form in countries such as Belgium, England, Germany and the Netherlands, and is increasing in several countries, such as Finland, Ireland, Italy and Slovakia. Privatization of home care puts governments at a larger distance. A supervisory role implies sufficient regulation to allow interference where quality of care or the position of clients is threatened, without harming the efficiency and flexibility expected as the benefits of privatization. Some experts mentioned a lack of regulation on private provision; others reported inefficiencies, lack of flexibility and higher costs resulting from overregulation. Finding the right balance is a major challenge in the home-care sector.

5.2.6 Enabling home care

In many cases formally provided home care is not an option if informal care is not available. There is still much to do in supporting informal carers, throughout Europe, but their acknowledgement as an essential element in home care has resulted in a range of regulation and arrangements to support informal care, including:

- cash payments to relatives and others who care for a dependent person
- training programmes for informal caregivers
- psychosocial counselling and general informational support
- social security benefits such as pension points.

they can set minimum requirements, monitor differences and influence local authorities.

5.2.3 Safeguarding coordination

Another typical feature of the home-care sector in almost all countries[1] is the different governance structures for the three streams of domestic aid, personal care and nursing care. This fragmented governance is a cause of poor coordination in cases that require more than one type of care. Social home care is decentralized more often than home health care. Additionally, national-level responsibility for social home care and home health care usually resides under different ministries and thus different legislation, regulations and financing schemes apply. As a consequence, the delivery of home health care and home social care may be poorly integrated. Overall, it may be concluded that coordination of home-care services is rather an exception than the rule. This could be tackled by investing in multiprofessional teamwork, an approach that has been shown to be successful.

Intersectoral coordination between home health care and hospitals is relatively well developed. Social workers and liaison nurses working in the context of protocols and agreements are important ingredients. However, such arrangements are not well developed between home care and nursing homes and there are lessons to be learned from the home care/hospital processes.

Nevertheless, in most countries, coordination between home care and other care providers – including hospitals – relates mainly to home health care rather than home social care. Positive exceptions are the Scandinavian countries where both types of services are also integrated at governance and provision levels. In addition to these countries, formal integration of home care and other health-care provision is best developed in England, the Netherlands and Slovakia.

5.2.4 'Marketing'

A cause of unmet needs in home care is the disconnection between demand and supply. Potential clients and even referring professionals may not be familiar with available home-care services. The visibility of home care may be improved by setting up a one-stop information window (either physically or on the Internet) for potential clients and carers and, at the same time, improving information to key referring providers (e.g. GPs, social workers, community nurses) or posting case managers between clients and the services.

---

1 Except Denmark, Greece, Sweden and some parts of Portugal and Finland.

As home care is largely decentralized, insight into the problems of the sector at central level is not optimal and will not be improved by the trend of increasing private home-care provision. Little is known about services provided by the privately financed sector; the quality of care; and the costs of its services, especially where care is purchased without any public intermediary. Additionally, personal budgets enable clients to purchase care, if so desired, from private or public providers and from professionals or non-professionals. The multitude of care options will make insight and, hence, quality control more complex. A comprehensive policy on home care should include a duty for governments to at least monitor services provided in the private sector and understand possible gaps between the publicly funded, regulated and privately funded subsectors. Policy-makers could consider introducing uniform reporting requirements on the care process for both the public and private sectors. Private providers may need to be more accountable for the number, type and education of professionals working in their agencies.

5.2.5 Balancing regulation, flexibility and efficiency

Currently, home care provided by private (profit-making or non-profit-making) agencies is the dominant form in countries such as Belgium, England, Germany and the Netherlands, and is increasing in several countries, such as Finland, Ireland, Italy and Slovakia. Privatization of home care puts governments at a larger distance. A supervisory role implies sufficient regulation to allow interference where quality of care or the position of clients is threatened, without harming the efficiency and flexibility expected as the benefits of privatization. Some experts mentioned a lack of regulation on private provision; others reported inefficiencies, lack of flexibility and higher costs resulting from overregulation. Finding the right balance is a major challenge in the home-care sector.

5.2.6 Enabling home care

In many cases formally provided home care is not an option if informal care is not available. There is still much to do in supporting informal carers, throughout Europe, but their acknowledgement as an essential element in home care has resulted in a range of regulation and arrangements to support informal care, including:

- cash payments to relatives and others who care for a dependent person
- training programmes for informal caregivers
- psychosocial counselling and general informational support
- social security benefits such as pension points.

they can set minimum requirements, monitor differences and influence local authorities.

5.2.3 Safeguarding coordination

Another typical feature of the home-care sector in almost all countries[1] is the different governance structures for the three streams of domestic aid, personal care and nursing care. This fragmented governance is a cause of poor coordination in cases that require more than one type of care. Social home care is decentralized more often than home health care. Additionally, national-level responsibility for social home care and home health care usually resides under different ministries and thus different legislation, regulations and financing schemes apply. As a consequence, the delivery of home health care and home social care may be poorly integrated. Overall, it may be concluded that coordination of home-care services is rather an exception than the rule. This could be tackled by investing in multiprofessional teamwork, an approach that has been shown to be successful.

Intersectoral coordination between home health care and hospitals is relatively well developed. Social workers and liaison nurses working in the context of protocols and agreements are important ingredients. However, such arrangements are not well developed between home care and nursing homes and there are lessons to be learned from the home care/hospital processes.

Nevertheless, in most countries, coordination between home care and other care providers – including hospitals – relates mainly to home health care rather than home social care. Positive exceptions are the Scandinavian countries where both types of services are also integrated at governance and provision levels. In addition to these countries, formal integration of home care and other health-care provision is best developed in England, the Netherlands and Slovakia.

5.2.4 'Marketing'

A cause of unmet needs in home care is the disconnection between demand and supply. Potential clients and even referring professionals may not be familiar with available home-care services. The visibility of home care may be improved by setting up a one-stop information window (either physically or on the Internet) for potential clients and carers and, at the same time, improving information to key referring providers (e.g. GPs, social workers, community nurses) or posting case managers between clients and the services.

---

1 Except Denmark, Greece, Sweden and some parts of Portugal and Finland.

As home care is largely decentralized, insight into the problems of the sector at central level is not optimal and will not be improved by the trend of increasing private home-care provision. Little is known about services provided by the privately financed sector; the quality of care; and the costs of its services, especially where care is purchased without any public intermediary. Additionally, personal budgets enable clients to purchase care, if so desired, from private or public providers and from professionals or non-professionals. The multitude of care options will make insight and, hence, quality control more complex. A comprehensive policy on home care should include a duty for governments to at least monitor services provided in the private sector and understand possible gaps between the publicly funded, regulated and privately funded subsectors. Policy-makers could consider introducing uniform reporting requirements on the care process for both the public and private sectors. Private providers may need to be more accountable for the number, type and education of professionals working in their agencies.

5.2.5 Balancing regulation, flexibility and efficiency

Currently, home care provided by private (profit-making or non-profit-making) agencies is the dominant form in countries such as Belgium, England, Germany and the Netherlands, and is increasing in several countries, such as Finland, Ireland, Italy and Slovakia. Privatization of home care puts governments at a larger distance. A supervisory role implies sufficient regulation to allow interference where quality of care or the position of clients is threatened, without harming the efficiency and flexibility expected as the benefits of privatization. Some experts mentioned a lack of regulation on private provision; others reported inefficiencies, lack of flexibility and higher costs resulting from overregulation. Finding the right balance is a major challenge in the home-care sector.

5.2.6 Enabling home care

In many cases formally provided home care is not an option if informal care is not available. There is still much to do in supporting informal carers, throughout Europe, but their acknowledgement as an essential element in home care has resulted in a range of regulation and arrangements to support informal care, including:

- cash payments to relatives and others who care for a dependent person
- training programmes for informal caregivers
- psychosocial counselling and general informational support
- social security benefits such as pension points.

they can set minimum requirements, monitor differences and influence local authorities.

5.2.3 Safeguarding coordination

Another typical feature of the home-care sector in almost all countries[1] is the different governance structures for the three streams of domestic aid, personal care and nursing care. This fragmented governance is a cause of poor coordination in cases that require more than one type of care. Social home care is decentralized more often than home health care. Additionally, national-level responsibility for social home care and home health care usually resides under different ministries and thus different legislation, regulations and financing schemes apply. As a consequence, the delivery of home health care and home social care may be poorly integrated. Overall, it may be concluded that coordination of home-care services is rather an exception than the rule. This could be tackled by investing in multiprofessional teamwork, an approach that has been shown to be successful.

Intersectoral coordination between home health care and hospitals is relatively well developed. Social workers and liaison nurses working in the context of protocols and agreements are important ingredients. However, such arrangements are not well developed between home care and nursing homes and there are lessons to be learned from the home care/hospital processes.

Nevertheless, in most countries, coordination between home care and other care providers – including hospitals – relates mainly to home health care rather than home social care. Positive exceptions are the Scandinavian countries where both types of services are also integrated at governance and provision levels. In addition to these countries, formal integration of home care and other health-care provision is best developed in England, the Netherlands and Slovakia.

5.2.4 'Marketing'

A cause of unmet needs in home care is the disconnection between demand and supply. Potential clients and even referring professionals may not be familiar with available home-care services. The visibility of home care may be improved by setting up a one-stop information window (either physically or on the Internet) for potential clients and carers and, at the same time, improving information to key referring providers (e.g. GPs, social workers, community nurses) or posting case managers between clients and the services.

---

[1] Except Denmark, Greece, Sweden and some parts of Portugal and Finland.

As home care is largely decentralized, insight into the problems of the sector at central level is not optimal and will not be improved by the trend of increasing private home-care provision. Little is known about services provided by the privately financed sector; the quality of care; and the costs of its services, especially where care is purchased without any public intermediary. Additionally, personal budgets enable clients to purchase care, if so desired, from private or public providers and from professionals or non-professionals. The multitude of care options will make insight and, hence, quality control more complex. A comprehensive policy on home care should include a duty for governments to at least monitor services provided in the private sector and understand possible gaps between the publicly funded, regulated and privately funded subsectors. Policy-makers could consider introducing uniform reporting requirements on the care process for both the public and private sectors. Private providers may need to be more accountable for the number, type and education of professionals working in their agencies.

5.2.5 Balancing regulation, flexibility and efficiency

Currently, home care provided by private (profit-making or non-profit-making) agencies is the dominant form in countries such as Belgium, England, Germany and the Netherlands, and is increasing in several countries, such as Finland, Ireland, Italy and Slovakia. Privatization of home care puts governments at a larger distance. A supervisory role implies sufficient regulation to allow interference where quality of care or the position of clients is threatened, without harming the efficiency and flexibility expected as the benefits of privatization. Some experts mentioned a lack of regulation on private provision; others reported inefficiencies, lack of flexibility and higher costs resulting from overregulation. Finding the right balance is a major challenge in the home-care sector.

5.2.6 Enabling home care

In many cases formally provided home care is not an option if informal care is not available. There is still much to do in supporting informal carers, throughout Europe, but their acknowledgement as an essential element in home care has resulted in a range of regulation and arrangements to support informal care, including:

- cash payments to relatives and others who care for a dependent person
- training programmes for informal caregivers
- psychosocial counselling and general informational support
- social security benefits such as pension points.

5.2.3 Safeguarding coordination

Another typical feature of the home-care sector in almost all countries[1] is the different governance structures for the three streams of domestic aid, personal care and nursing care. This fragmented governance is a cause of poor coordination in cases that require more than one type of care. Social home care is decentralized more often than home health care. Additionally, national-level responsibility for social home care and home health care usually resides under different ministries and thus different legislation, regulations and financing schemes apply. As a consequence, the delivery of home health care and home social care may be poorly integrated. Overall, it may be concluded that coordination of home-care services is rather an exception than the rule. This could be tackled by investing in multiprofessional teamwork, an approach that has been shown to be successful.

Intersectoral coordination between home health care and hospitals is relatively well developed. Social workers and liaison nurses working in the context of protocols and agreements are important ingredients. However, such arrangements are not well developed between home care and nursing homes and there are lessons to be learned from the home care/hospital processes.

Nevertheless, in most countries, coordination between home care and other care providers – including hospitals – relates mainly to home health care rather than home social care. Positive exceptions are the Scandinavian countries where both types of services are also integrated at governance and provision levels. In addition to these countries, formal integration of home care and other health-care provision is best developed in England, the Netherlands and Slovakia.

5.2.4 'Marketing'

A cause of unmet needs in home care is the disconnection between demand and supply. Potential clients and even referring professionals may not be familiar with available home-care services. The visibility of home care may be improved by setting up a one-stop information window (either physically or on the Internet) for potential clients and carers and, at the same time, improving information to key referring providers (e.g. GPs, social workers, community nurses) or posting case managers between clients and the services.

---

1 Except Denmark, Greece, Sweden and some parts of Portugal and Finland.

As home care is largely decentralized, insight into the problems of the sector at central level is not optimal and will not be improved by the trend of increasing private home-care provision. Little is known about services provided by the privately financed sector; the quality of care; and the costs of its services, especially where care is purchased without any public intermediary. Additionally, personal budgets enable clients to purchase care, if so desired, from private or public providers and from professionals or non-professionals. The multitude of care options will make insight and, hence, quality control more complex. A comprehensive policy on home care should include a duty for governments to at least monitor services provided in the private sector and understand possible gaps between the publicly funded, regulated and privately funded subsectors. Policy-makers could consider introducing uniform reporting requirements on the care process for both the public and private sectors. Private providers may need to be more accountable for the number, type and education of professionals working in their agencies.

5.2.5 Balancing regulation, flexibility and efficiency

Currently, home care provided by private (profit-making or non-profit-making) agencies is the dominant form in countries such as Belgium, England, Germany and the Netherlands, and is increasing in several countries, such as Finland, Ireland, Italy and Slovakia. Privatization of home care puts governments at a larger distance. A supervisory role implies sufficient regulation to allow interference where quality of care or the position of clients is threatened, without harming the efficiency and flexibility expected as the benefits of privatization. Some experts mentioned a lack of regulation on private provision; others reported inefficiencies, lack of flexibility and higher costs resulting from overregulation. Finding the right balance is a major challenge in the home-care sector.

5.2.6 Enabling home care

In many cases formally provided home care is not an option if informal care is not available. There is still much to do in supporting informal carers, throughout Europe, but their acknowledgement as an essential element in home care has resulted in a range of regulation and arrangements to support informal care, including:

- cash payments to relatives and others who care for a dependent person
- training programmes for informal caregivers
- psychosocial counselling and general informational support
- social security benefits such as pension points.

they can set minimum requirements, monitor differences and influence local authorities.

5.2.3 Safeguarding coordination

Another typical feature of the home-care sector in almost all countries[1] is the different governance structures for the three streams of domestic aid, personal care and nursing care. This fragmented governance is a cause of poor coordination in cases that require more than one type of care. Social home care is decentralized more often than home health care. Additionally, national-level responsibility for social home care and home health care usually resides under different ministries and thus different legislation, regulations and financing schemes apply. As a consequence, the delivery of home health care and home social care may be poorly integrated. Overall, it may be concluded that coordination of home-care services is rather an exception than the rule. This could be tackled by investing in multiprofessional teamwork, an approach that has been shown to be successful.

Intersectoral coordination between home health care and hospitals is relatively well developed. Social workers and liaison nurses working in the context of protocols and agreements are important ingredients. However, such arrangements are not well developed between home care and nursing homes and there are lessons to be learned from the home care/hospital processes.

Nevertheless, in most countries, coordination between home care and other care providers – including hospitals – relates mainly to home health care rather than home social care. Positive exceptions are the Scandinavian countries where both types of services are also integrated at governance and provision levels. In addition to these countries, formal integration of home care and other health-care provision is best developed in England, the Netherlands and Slovakia.

5.2.4 'Marketing'

A cause of unmet needs in home care is the disconnection between demand and supply. Potential clients and even referring professionals may not be familiar with available home-care services. The visibility of home care may be improved by setting up a one-stop information window (either physically or on the Internet) for potential clients and carers and, at the same time, improving information to key referring providers (e.g. GPs, social workers, community nurses) or posting case managers between clients and the services.

---

1 Except Denmark, Greece, Sweden and some parts of Portugal and Finland.

As home care is largely decentralized, insight into the problems of the sector at central level is not optimal and will not be improved by the trend of increasing private home-care provision. Little is known about services provided by the privately financed sector; the quality of care; and the costs of its services, especially where care is purchased without any public intermediary. Additionally, personal budgets enable clients to purchase care, if so desired, from private or public providers and from professionals or non-professionals. The multitude of care options will make insight and, hence, quality control more complex. A comprehensive policy on home care should include a duty for governments to at least monitor services provided in the private sector and understand possible gaps between the publicly funded, regulated and privately funded subsectors. Policy-makers could consider introducing uniform reporting requirements on the care process for both the public and private sectors. Private providers may need to be more accountable for the number, type and education of professionals working in their agencies.

5.2.5 Balancing regulation, flexibility and efficiency

Currently, home care provided by private (profit-making or non-profit-making) agencies is the dominant form in countries such as Belgium, England, Germany and the Netherlands, and is increasing in several countries, such as Finland, Ireland, Italy and Slovakia. Privatization of home care puts governments at a larger distance. A supervisory role implies sufficient regulation to allow interference where quality of care or the position of clients is threatened, without harming the efficiency and flexibility expected as the benefits of privatization. Some experts mentioned a lack of regulation on private provision; others reported inefficiencies, lack of flexibility and higher costs resulting from overregulation. Finding the right balance is a major challenge in the home-care sector.

5.2.6 Enabling home care

In many cases formally provided home care is not an option if informal care is not available. There is still much to do in supporting informal carers, throughout Europe, but their acknowledgement as an essential element in home care has resulted in a range of regulation and arrangements to support informal care, including:

- cash payments to relatives and others who care for a dependent person
- training programmes for informal caregivers
- psychosocial counselling and general informational support
- social security benefits such as pension points.

What is now labelled as informal care has always existed as the main source of help to elderly and ill people. Now, informal care is being preserved, promoted and increasingly formalized and integrated in formal home-care arrangements. Strengthening informal care means strengthening the basis for home care. Investments in informal-care support pay off not only in home care but also through wider social implications – it may prevent informal carers from becoming overburdened and then forced to rely completely on formal services and support.

Suitable housing is another precondition which is often lacking although home adaptations are funded in countries with more generous home-care schemes. Nevertheless, in some countries where there has been a reduction in residential care places (or a policy move to effect this), investment in new forms of living accommodation has been developed to assist independent living in a supported environment. This may prove to be a model for care for the future.

Improved technology is a relatively new enabling factor in home care, presenting both a promise and a challenge. Alarm buttons are used widely; telecare applications (such as video networks) are in their infancy today but look promising. Technology has the potential both to offer people opportunities to stay independent for longer in their homes and to make major steps forward in the efficient provision of home-care services. The challenge of technological innovation in the home-care sector is that, in times of financial constraints, policy-makers will need to make important investments before the potential becomes reality.

European countries have responded (or intend to respond) in various ways to the challenges they face in their home-care sectors. These responses have been summarized in Table 5.1, including their possible consequences for the costs, equity or quality of home care.

5.3 System-tailored responses to challenges

As care for people living at home is formalized and organized so differently across Europe, current challenges are felt differently and responses to the challenges are not similar. Home care in eastern and southern Europe is organized and provided more informally than, for instance, in Scandinavia, where publicly financed and provided home care is much more extensively available. The current economic situation may force countries with well resourced public home-care schemes to make these less generous. In countries where home care absorbs fewer public financial resources it may be that the sustainability of home-care schemes will be less of an issue. In the current economic downturn, countries may seek more inspiration from systems that rely relatively strongly on informal arrangements.

Table 5.1 Challenges in home care: responses and their possible consequences

Challenges	Responses (examples of countries where applied or planned)	Consequences to be taken into account
Access		
Poor accessibility	• 'one-stop' information windows (NL, DE) • preventive home visits (FI)	• increased demand • costs • need for extra coordination
Inequity (in quality; extent of delivery; and access)	• progressive financing system or basic insurance (HR, SK, LV) • general standards and requirements at national level and monitoring effectiveness (SI, SE)	• costs • eroding public support for system (solidarity) • lower flexibility and quality of care
Supply		
Few services available	• increasing public and/or private provision of home (nursing) care (19 countries) • specialized services at home (LU) • nongovernmental providers (profit-making or non-profit-making) entering home-care sector to provide additional services (BG) • new funding mechanisms to secure financing of home care (ES, EE, LV, PL, IT) • introduction of insured basic package of services (RO) • voluntary insurance for extra services (CH, HR, SI)	• costs • lower quality of care
Shortage of human resources	• shorter education pathways and lower educational requirements (LV, LU) • personal budgets (NL, EN, LV) • paying migrant workers' pension benefits (AU) • paying relatives; paying informal caregivers' state pension benefits (CY, IT, CZ, DE, AU) • task delegation from higher-skilled to lower-skilled workers (DK, NL, BE, FI) • telecare (LU) • stimulating and supporting informal caregiving (most countries)	• costs • objections of professionals • lower quality of care • migration and resulting problems
Shortage of providers	• expanding the number of professionals (BG, SK) • stimulating private provision (IR, FI)	• costs (long-term) • lower quality of care
Problems related to migrant workers	• formalizing carers in the 'informal circuit' (AU, CY)	• migration and resulting problems • costs

Table 5.1 contd

Challenges	Responses (examples of countries where applied or planned)	Consequences to be taken into account
Quality		
Variation in quality of care	• (additional) educational requirements (BG, CY) • quality certification for care providers (NL) • quality control mechanisms (BE, GR, DE). • official national 'frameworks' for quality (FI, EN, NL, LU) • publishing quality performances of providers (NL, DK, EN, DE) • investing in the client-centredness of home care (DK, DE, EN) • complaints procedures (BG, SK, HU, PT)	• costs of monitoring • lack of flexibility, lower quality • need for extra coordination
Funding		
Poor funding	• new financing mechanisms (LV, PL; corresponding plans in DE) • childless people make higher contributions to long-term care insurance (DE) • competition among providers (NL, EN, IR) • client co-payments/means testing for middle class and for higher earners (RO) • transparency of costs (FI, NL, HR) • rationing services (most countries) • preventive home visits (FI) • group approaches: supportive communities (CZ) • increasing efficiency (LV, CH)	• costs • lower quality • more pressure on informal carers
No earmarked budget for home care	• transparency in health and social care budgets (NL)	• costs
Unfair differentiation in payments	• payment related to case load; case mix; quality (BE, EN)	• costs
Lack of (national) regulation	• quality control over providers (NO) • centralized decision-making (FR, CY) • more transparency of expenditures on home care (NL)	• costs • danger of overregulation
Integration		
Poor integration of different types of home care	• interdisciplinary teamwork (NL, IR, IT) • defining roles and boundaries of health/nursing care and social care/domestic aid (EN) • financing of coordination time (BE)	• costs

Table 5.1 contd

Challenges	Responses (examples of countries where applied or planned)	Consequences to be taken into account
Integration		
Poor integration with nursing homes and hospitals	• liaison nurses for hospital discharge (NL, ES) • case managers for clients with chronic conditions (BE, EN) • transmural networks or teams (FI, BE, NL) • common electronic client record systems (FI)	• costs

AU: Austria; BE: Belgium; BG: Bulgaria; CH: Switzerland; CY: Cyprus; CZ: Czech Republic; DE: Germany; DK: Denmark; EE: Estonia; EN: England; ES: Spain; FI: Finland; FR: France; GR: Greece; HR: Croatia; HU: Hungary; IR: Ireland; IT: Italy; LU: Luxembourg; LV: Latvia; NL: the Netherlands; NO: Norway; PL: Poland; PT: Portugal; RO: Romania; SE: Sweden; SI: Slovenia; SK: Slovakia.

Table 5.2 aims to show that well resourced and less well resourced countries have not only different problems but also different options to solve them. The two types of country have been divided further into three categories of funding of home-care schemes: (i) completely publicly funded and provided; (ii) largely privately provided and funded; and (iii) mixed systems (see Table 5.2).

In the group of countries with well resourced and mainly publicly financed and provided services (indicated with *(1)* in Table 5.2), home care is largely decentralized and there is currently a lower level of unmet need. The relatively high expenditures on care are being discussed in these countries. Concerns about sustainability have grown due to the current recession, decreasing tax and social contribution base and growing demand. Under such circumstances these countries may opt for cost containment measures (e.g. reducing services being funded, investing in preventive services, increasing client co-payments or increasing efficiency through reorganization of services). Areas differ slightly in the means testing of home-care benefits but generally no, or only a modest, co-payment is needed for home health care. However, this may change in the future.

In countries with mainly privately financed or provided home care (*(2)* in Table 5.2), concerns about the sustainability of current systems, client empowerment and lack of regulation of private provision seem to be major points of discussion. Options for change may be to introduce more regulation on privately funded agencies and to increase quality by investing in client empowerment. In such a context, clients should have adequate skills to purchase care and to evaluate the provision of private care purchased outside the public sector or bought through personal budgets. However, this will require caution with regulation as lessons from other countries point to the risk of overregulation. Privately provided care

Table 5.2 *Typology of home-care systems: different challenges and solutions*

Type of country	Mode of funding/provision of home care		
	Public	**Mixed public-private**	**Private**
	Explanation		
Financially well resourced	Extensive publicly financed and provided home care *(1)*	Obligatory insurance and mainly private provision but strong governmental regulation *(2)*	Low public financing; clients make large direct or co-payments; provision mainly by private organizations *(3)*
	Challenges		
	Expenditures too high	Cost of regulation and monitoring; little control of expenditures on home care; home-care profession has little attraction	Quality & equity problems (access to public funding) as no insight into the provision of private organizations
	Options		
	Increasing private sector provision and financing; supporting informal care; more efficient ways of provision	Supporting informal care and efficient provision; decreasing regulation by incentives for self-regulation; introduction of personal budget instead of benefits in kind	More regulation on privately funded and provided organizations and client empowerment
	Explanation		
Financially less well resourced	Acts as 'safety net' for poorest and those without children; public services provided for free or low payment *(4)*	Coverage by obligatory insurance; mainly private provision *(5)*	Out-of-pocket either direct payments or lost income due to care duties; professional care provided mainly by NGO *(6)*
	Challenges		
	Gaps between privately and publicly financed services; informal caregivers overburdened; informal caregivers; maintaining public support once economic conditions improve	When available resources grow, grip on expenditures may become problematic	Affordable home care; quality control absent; lack of informal and formal care
	Options		
	Support informal care; increase funding for other socioeconomic groups	Spending more on home care; more regulation and client empowerment	Safety net to larger groups or insurance coverage of home care; education of professionals

is not necessarily a threat to quality but little is known about the performance of this sector.

Home care in the Netherlands and Germany is characterized by a mix of private and public funding and primarily private provision under strict governmental regulation. In mixed systems ((2) in Table 5.2) overregulation, little control of expenditures and a lack of home-care professionals are important issues. These can be tackled by supporting informal care (e.g. through respite care, psychosocial help and training); stimulating efficient ways of provision (e.g. small-scale teams of professionals); and decreasing regulation by incentives for positive self-regulation of private organizations (providers, financers etc.). Each of these has its own disadvantages that need to be taken into account.

Support of new, less expensive, providers will become central to policies in countries with current high levels of public financial resources. Policy-makers may consider supporting informal care provision. For instance, introduce further institutionalization and integration of informal care by recognizing the role of informal caregivers; coordinating care between informal and formal carers; providing financial compensation; and providing a platform where volunteers can meet with those who need help. An alternative approach is to reduce the costs of service provision by encouraging competition among private providers. This is practised by many countries.

Ways need to be found to 'reach' the current workforce of migrant workers. They play a substantial role in home care in some countries. Migrant workers should be supported with training in both professional skills and, if necessary, language skills.

Other issues may arise in countries with fewer financial resources. Limited formal care may result from the general state of the economy but also from a cultural context in which informal care is preferred. However, migration within and between countries is causing informal caregivers to become scarcer, particularly in rural areas where the needs of ageing populations are high. Policy-makers in these countries may consider measures to promote and support informal care and prevent overburdening informal caregivers – for instance, through education and training and by offering respite care.

In most of the countries with fewer financial resources, a home-care policy has been developed but the allocation of resources lags behind. Public funding and the provision of home care serves mainly as a safety net for the most disadvantaged (those with lowest income, severe disabilities and no relatives) ((4) in Table 5.2). Safety-net schemes are found in Bulgaria and Romania. Public systems in these countries may be complemented not only by systems funded and provided by charitable organizations but also by services funded through direct payments or private insurance ((6) in Table 5.2). Access to home-care services is not limited simply by financial barriers; many people do not know about the existence of home care. In these countries, the first steps to improve home-care delivery could be expansion of the safety-net function.

Among the countries that are less well resourced ((5) in Table 5.2), mixed systems are found where there is an intermediate level of public funding of home care, together with insurance-based funding and private provision. These are found mainly in the home health-care sector within eastern European countries such as Slovakia and Hungary. Private professional care is quite new in these countries. Sustainable funding poses a major challenge, as does controlling expenditures and safeguarding information for clients. There is a need to empower clients and to develop regulation to ensure affordable and good quality of care. Countries with sparsely populated areas have an additional challenge to safeguard good service provision in remote areas. Integration and task substitution may help to enable single professionals to combine different types of services and thus reduce travelling time and costs.

Countries with similar home-care systems, facing comparable challenges, may learn from one another's solutions and best practices as well as the pitfalls and mistakes. However, in times of austerity, countries with larger financial resources can also be inspired by the experiences of countries with fewer resources – for instance, how to target those most in need and new ways of organizing provision. Useful lessons can also be learned about efficient organization of service delivery (especially regarding private providers) and to identify and involve new home-care resources, such as alternative providers or informal caregivers. New arrangements can be designed by smart combinations of public and private initiatives, of formal and informal care.

All countries will face a major challenge in adapting to the expected decline in the availability of informal caregivers. Investment to reduce the burden of informal care and to make the choice of becoming an informal caregiver more attractive will be needed and should eventually turn out to be beneficial. The ageing of Europe's populations is not just a reason for concern; it is also an opportunity. Most of today's younger elderly remain vital, looking for meaningful activities in their spare time. Shared informal care can become a serious option if supporting conditions are in place. Thinking beyond the borders of health and social care may bring solutions for home-care problems closer. The need for intersectoral action will grow.

5.4 Ways forward: the EU perspective

The EURHOMAP study has been co-financed by the European Commission. Indeed, the EU has a role in home care even though it is primarily the national responsibility of Member States. Where common challenges can be identified and countries are open to learn from foreign experiences, the European Commission can establish a source of information and a platform for exchange. The provision of sound and comparable information on home care in European countries fits well with this role and is where this book makes its main contribution. The EURHOMAP project (including this book and the publicly accessible database as the main product) has promoted the systematic gathering of information all over Europe, resulting not only in a wealth of comparable data on the home-care sector but also identifying the sources (and lack) of information in each country and the many experts that were able to provide the details and realities behind statistics and policy papers. Not surprisingly, the comparability of data left something to be desired and, in the absence of hard data, expert opinions had to be accepted instead. Furthermore, available information sometimes lacked detail, or evident regional variation within a country could not be taken fully into account. In what it describes, and by its omissions, this book reflects the current diversity in available information on the home-care sector in Europe. The infrastructure developed through this project could be used to improve this situation and to work towards more detailed and more comparable updates.

Some general problems and challenges in the home-care sector may require action at a European level. One example of this is the unfavourable working conditions of personal carers and domestic assistants in several countries, which are among the reasons for current staff shortages in home care. These shortages are expected to increase. Furthermore, the home-care sector could benefit from joint action by Member States and some harmonization of national regulation and procedures.

The European Commission could also encourage Member States to develop innovative housing for specific target groups, such as people with physical disabilities; housing for families that want to care for their elderly parents; and independent group-housing for elderly people.

5.5 Options for policy-makers

For national governments

- To better inform clients about where and how to apply for home care, what services are available and under what conditions. This is a major concern throughout Europe and is relevant for potential clients and for health and social-care professionals. Possible solutions include setting up a (digital) one-stop information window; introduction of case managers; and briefing referring care professionals (e.g. GP, social worker, community nurse) about details and changes in the system.

- To introduce at national level minimum standards on eligibility and quality of care. Geographical differences in home care due to decentralization demand better control of home-care provision, particularly in countries where financing has been decentralized (partly or completely) to local governments.

- To better understand and find proper ways to regulate the growing private sector. At present there is little control over access to, and the quality of, privately financed home-care services. Furthermore, knowledge about the availability of privately financed home care in a country is often lacking. As the importance of privately paid services grows, protection of clients could be a governmental role.

- To invest in client empowerment. Where clients are required to purchase their own home-care services (either through personal budgets or out-of-pocket) they should be able to negotiate with providers on the care that will be provided and to evaluate the quality of care. This will often require professional assistance.

- To support multiprofessional teamwork in home care. Experience has shown that small-scale provision is likely to be better and more efficient.

- To invest in telecare in order to achieve necessary gains in efficiency and to decrease unmet needs, especially in remote areas.

- To promote and enable informal care through (partial) financial compensation and to develop arrangements to facilitate multigenerational living.

- To promote life-proof housing in which people with reduced mobility are able to live longer independently in adapted houses.

For the European Commission

- To encourage Member States to obtain more insight into their home-care sectors. More, as well as more comparable, data should be gathered on home-care recipients, unmet needs, expenditures, numbers and types of home care professionals, at both national and regional level. This will allow countries to learn from foreign experiences.

- To support sustainability of home-care systems. Home-care schemes in several countries have been supported by EU structural funds. Some countries had problems with continuity when this funding stopped. Attention should be paid to safeguarding continued financing in such situations.

- To improve working conditions for social home-care workers. Unfavourable working conditions may further aggravate the current lack of human resources in personal care and domestic aid.

5.6 In conclusion

Home care is in demand, not only among citizens in Europe (who prefer to stay independent as long as possible), but also among decision-makers (who expect it to be a cheaper alternative to hospital-based and nursing home care). In most countries, demand for home care cannot yet be met by the available formal home-care schemes; in a number of countries home-care policy is not well articulated. Policies and regulation have been formulated but still need to be fully implemented. Ambitions to develop and expand the home-care sector in European countries will be difficult to realize in a time of severe financial constraints and unconventional solutions will need to be tried to bridge the gap between growing need and shrinking budgets. Retreating governments and the growing role of the private sector may drive a need to find a new balance between the regulation, efficiency and flexibility of service delivery. However, some principles should not be compromised. Frail dependent people need to be protected against quality failures and unaffordable care. And, in general, better client information and empowerment should become more important. To find solutions in response to these challenges, policy-makers will need to look for inspiration beyond the usual models and good practices. The descriptions in this book are an entry point to ideas from other countries.

Appendix I
Terminology

Activities of daily living (ADL): both personal activities of daily living (PADL) and instrumental activities of daily living (IADL).

Delivery: activities organized within public and privately owned agencies and institutions which are meant to deliver social and health-care services in clients' homes.

Domestic aid: help with instrumental activities of daily living (IADL), such as using the telephone, shopping, food preparation, housekeeping, transportation, taking medication and financial administration.[1]

Financing: process by which revenue is collected from primary and secondary sources, accumulated in fund pools and allocated to provider priorities.

Governance: policy development, supervision of a good functioning of the system and regulation to steer where necessary.

Home care: care provided at home by professionals after a formal needs assessment. 'Care' means domestic aid services, personal care and supportive, technical and rehabilitative nursing.

Home-care system: an integrated and interdependent set of elements that produce actions with the primary purpose of allowing people to live at home despite functional disabilities. Its functions are 'governance', 'financing', 'service delivery', 'needs assessment', 'safeguarding the quality of services' and 'human resources'.

Home health care: technical, supportive and rehabilitative services and possibly personal-care services depending on the characteristics and boundaries of both systems in a country.

Informal care: care provided by family members, friends and volunteers, usually unpaid.

---

1 Lawton MP, Brody EM (1969). Assessment of older people: self-maintaining and instrumental activities of daily living. *Gerontologist*, 9(3):179–186.

Instrumental activities of daily living (IADL): help with IADL relates to services such as assistance with using the telephone, shopping, food preparation, housekeeping, transportation, taking medication and financial administration.

Needs assessment: systematic exploration of the physical and financial possibilities of a person living independently, according to specified rules.

Nursing: activities of nurses that are of a technical, supportive or rehabilitative nature (see rehabilitative nursing, supportive nursing, technical nursing).

Personal activities of daily living (PADL): help with PADL relates to services such as assistance with dressing, feeding, washing and toileting, and getting in or out of bed.

Personal care services: providing assistance with dressing, feeding, washing and toileting, and getting in or out of bed (also known as PADL).

Privately/publicly funded organizations/services: providers or the activities of home-care services that are funded through tax revenue or social insurance (publicly funded) or *only* through a person's or his/her family's own financial resources or through private insurance schemes (privately funded).

Privately/publicly owned organizations: organizations that are legally owned mostly by the government (publicly owned) or by other organizations (privately owned).

Rehabilitative nursing: occupational therapy or physiotherapy.

Respite care: short-term care (e.g. help with ADL) aiming to relieve informal caregivers, i.e. providing the caregiver with time away from the patient.

Social home care: domestic aid and (depending on the country's system) personal care services.

Supportive nursing: provision of health information and education.

Technical nursing: Activities such as assistance with putting on prostheses or elastic stockings; changing stomas and urinal bags; help with bladder catheter/catheterization; skin care; disinfection and prevention of bedsores; oxygen administration; and giving intravenous injections.

Appendix II
Case narratives (vignettes)

Accompanying letter for the experts

Dear Madam, Sir,

We are glad with your preparedness to contribute to this European home care study. The study aims to describe and compare the organization and provision of home care services in Europe. One of the approaches to gather information is based on *vignettes*, which are (hypothetical) descriptions of situations of elderly or disabled people living at home in need of care. In all European countries, experts are asked to answer the questions related to two vignettes. Comparison of the answers will show the diversity of home care in the countries of Europe, in particular from a user's perspective.

Some of the questions to the vignettes can be answered by simply ticking a box, while others are open-ended. Since we attach great value on explanations that further clarify the situation in your country, you are encouraged to use the possibilities to expand on your answers or attach an annex to this questionnaire.

If you would not know an answer, you can tick the option 'I do not know' or, in case of open questions, just move on to the next question.

As a check of the information, the draft report concerning your country will be fed back to you.

For all your questions, please contact one of the undersigned people.

Thank you very much for your cooperation in this important study.

Name(s) from Eurhomap partner ………………………………. ……………………………….	Wienke Boerma (w.boerma@nivel.nl) Nadine Genet (n.genet@nivel.nl) Research Institute NIVEL (Netherlands) (www.nivel.eu)

If you would like to be acknowledged in the country report, please provide your details here:

Name:

Function:

Organization:

Address:

Vignette 1

Background
A couple, both 84, are physically relatively healthy, but the wife has symptoms of early stage dementia which is an increasing obstacle in her management of the household. For years they have hired a cleaning lady on a private basis twice a week, who also helps with preparing meals. The children are committed and give support as far as possible beside their jobs and other obligations. One daughter with 3 children under the age of 20 is living nearby, while another, widowed with two grown up children, and a single son are living at half an hour travel distance.

What happened
The lady falls and breaks her hip. She is hospitalized for an operation and subsequently admitted to a nursing home for recovery and initial rehabilitation. Her situation develops well and returning home, which is her preferred option, is possible if precautionary measures are taken. Measures should also focus on safety issues related to expected increase of dementia problems.

Care needs
At home, at least for some time, she will need help getting up, washing herself and going to bed. Furthermore, the lady will temporarily need continued rehabilitation to further improve walking. Since she will no longer be able to oversee household and daily activities, more help will be needed for cleaning the home, shopping and preparing meals. Timely intake of medicines should also be taken care of. Since there is no bathroom at the ground floor of the house, a solution needs to be found for her to get upstairs.

(Format of the questionnaire has been slightly compressed)

Please answer the following questions

1.1 To what home care services would this lady be entitled <u>according to current criteria and rules</u> in your country (so, this is about the 'theory'; the practice may be different!).
She is <u>entitled</u> to the following services:
………………………………………………………………………………..

1.2 Which of the needs of this lady would be covered by the services for which she is ('theoretically') entitled, and for which of her needs other solutions should be found (or remain unmet)?
Entitled services cover the following needs of the lady:
………………………………………………………………………………..

The following needs cannot be met according to rules of entitlement
....

1.3 Do financial consequences for the client apply to the acceptance of the eligible services in this case (for instance co-payments or other financial contributions)? *(please explain)*
....

1.4 Does a gap exist between the services to which the lady is entitled and the services she will effectively receive? (This gap may result from possible shortages and other imperfections in your country).
(*You may tick more than one box*)
- ❏ Normally all services to which she is entitled will be provided without reduction
- ❏ Usually, reductions are applied (for instance in number of hours of care) in the provision of the following type(s) of services. *Please fill in:*
....
- ❏ Usually the following type(s) of services are not available at all. *Please, fill in:*
....
- ❏ I do not know

Please further explain your answer:
....

1.5 Would some telecare application be used in this situation in your country? (Examples of telecare are personal alarm systems, distant observations and other ICT applications in home care). *(please tick the most applicable box)*
- ❏ No tele-care applications will be used in this case
- ❏ Yes, the following telecare applications can be used (also indicate the probability of use)
  1. (fill in a telecare application): ....
     How often will this be used in cases like this? *(tick a box)*
     ❏ often ❏ occasionally ❏ infrequent / rarely

  2. (fill in another application, if applicable): ....
     How often will this be used in cases like this? *(tick a box)*
     ❏ often ❏ occasionally ❏ infrequent / rarely

  3. (fill in another application, if applicable): ....
     How often will this be used in cases like this? *(tick a box)*
     ❏ often ❏ occasionally ❏ infrequent / rarely
- ❏ I do not know

Please further explain your answer:
....

1.6 In your country, who would most probably take the initiative in this case to apply for care? *(please tick the most applicable box)*
- ❏ The couple or family
- ❏ The nursing home
- ❏ The GP of the couple

❑ Someone else, namely *(fill in)*: ....
❑ It depends on the situation who will take the initiative *(please explain below)*
❑ I do not know
Please further explain your answer:
....

1.7 In your country, is there usually 'one window' for all services relevant to this application for care (as the start of the care process) or are different bodies to be approached separately? *(please tick the most appropriate box)*
❑ There is one window or entry point for all home care services needed
❑ Each service has its own entry point
❑ The situation is different, namely *(please fill in)*: ....
❑ I do not know
Please further explain your answer:
....

1.8 Who will usually <u>assess the needs</u> and the personal situation of the lady? Needs assessment is done by:
❑ An independent formal assessing agency
❑ A representative of the home care provider
❑ A governmental organization
❑ Another type of organization, namely: ....
❑ It depends
❑ I do not know.
Please explain your answer:
....

1.9 Are explicit (written and publicly known) <u>eligibility criteria</u> used in needs assessment in this case? *(please, tick the most appropriate box)*
❑ In this case nationwide used criteria are applied
❑ Criteria are used, but these are not used everywhere and not uniformly
❑ No explicit criteria will be used
❑ Another situation, namely *(please fill in)*:
....
❑ I do not know
Please further explain your answer:
....

1.10 In your country, who would take the <u>decision</u> about the granting of the requested services?
The granting decision will be taken by:
....

1.11 In this case, will the <u>availability of informal carers</u> (children) be taken into consideration in the decision to grant services? If yes, in which way? *(please, tick the most appropriate box)*
❑ No, the availability of informal care is not taken into consideration
❑ Yes, availability of informal care is taken into consideration, as follows:

(please fill in):
....
❏ I do not know

1.12 In this case, will the <u>financial situation</u> of the couple be taken into consideration in the decision to grant services? If yes, in which way? *(please, tick the most appropriate box)*
❏ No, the financial situation is not taken into consideration
❏ Yes, the financial situation is taken into consideration, as follows: *(please fill in):*
....
❏ I do not know

1.13 Which care providers (professional and other) will probably be involved in home care for the couple? (*You may tick more than one answer*)
❏ Home help (domestic aid)
❏ Nurse
❏ Social worker
❏ Physiotherapist
❏ Occupational therapist
❏ Family doctor
❏ Children of the couple
❏ Volunteers
❏ Neighbours
❏ Friends
❏ Others, namely *(please fill in)*: ....
❏ I do not know
Please further explain your answer:
....

1.14 Will the process of care to this couple be explicitly <u>monitored</u> from time to time to assess whether the provided care is still appropriate in relation to the couple's needs? ('explicitly' meaning that it is done by a formal procedure at regular intervals) *(please tick one box)*
❏ Services to this couple will not be explicitly monitored (monitoring procedures do not exist in this country)
❏ Services to this couple will not be explicitly monitored (existing procedures are not widely used)
❏ Services to this couple will be monitored according to an explicit systematic procedure
❏ I do not know
Please further explain your answer (including who will do the monitoring):
....

1.15 If, in your country, formal home care would probably <u>not</u> be an option to this couple, what would likely be their situation or what would be the solution? *(you may tick more boxes, but limit to 'most probable')*
❏ Not applicable, because home care is the most likely option in this case

- ❏ The lady would be in a home for the elderly (separated from her husband)
- ❏ The couple would be in a home for the elderly
- ❏ The couple would live with one of the children
- ❏ The widowed daughter would reduce her job to care for them
- ❏ The couple would hire private care (paying 'black')
- ❏ The couple would hire private care (paying tax etc.)
- ❏ The couple would suffer from unmet needs (health and social threats)
- ❏ Another situation, namely *(please fill in):*
  ....
- ❏ I do not know

Please further explain your answer (and distinguish which of the children would have which role)
....

1.16 Related to the situation and the needs of this couple, what are frequently occurring difficulties, possible unmet care needs or other peculiarities, if they lived in your country? Would it make a difference in home care for them to live in a city or in a rural area?
Please explain the possible difficulties, peculiarities or differences:
....

Vignette 2

Background
A 91-year-old widow is living independently in a single family dwelling. None of her six children, two of which are retired, is living nearby. She is getting her meals from a meals-on-wheels service. Once a week a privately hired cleaning lady is doing domestic work. Additional care is provided by her children on a rota basis.

What happened
Her major health problem is increasing poor walking, which restricts her mobility and ability to cope with daily living and household tasks. Even in-house she cannot walk without a Zimmer frame (rollator). Going up and down the stairs is becoming extremely difficult. Sometimes she is found to be slovenly and she sometimes has problems structuring her days, especially at occasions when she has taken too much alcohol. The only formal care she receives is the occasional home visits from her GP, with whom she has good contact. Since the situation is expected to further deteriorate and the children feel they are at the limit of their possibilities, they all agree that measures need to be taken.

Care needs
Institutionalization is no solution, since she strongly wants to stay at home. Having her bed in the living room and building a basic bathroom facility on the ground floor would make the use of the upper floor superfluous. Besides, on working days she would need help with getting up, washing and dressing and getting to bed. Since she is unable to clean the house and shop, more support will be needed for these tasks.

(Format of the questionnaire has been slightly compressed)

Please answer the following questions

2.1 To what home care services would this lady be entitled <u>according to current criteria and rules</u> in your country (so, this is about the 'theory'; the practice may be different!) (also consider the bathing facility).
She is <u>entitled</u> to the following services:
....

2.2 Which of the needs of this lady would be covered by the services for which she is ('theoretically') entitled, and for which of her needs other solutions should be found (or remain unmet)?
Entitled services cover the following needs of the lady:
....

The following needs cannot be met according to rules of entitlement
....

2.3 Do financial consequences for the client apply to the acceptance of the eligible services in this case (for instance co-payments or other financial contributions)? *(please explain)*

2.4 Does a gap exist between the services to which the lady is entitled and the services she will effectively receive? (This gap may result from possible shortages and other imperfections in your country).
 (You may tick more than one box)
 ❏ Normally all services to which she is entitled will be provided without reduction
 ❏ Usually, reductions are applied (for instance in number of hours of care) in the provision of the following type(s) of services.
 Please fill in:
 ....
 ❏ Usually the following type(s) of services are not available at all.
 Please, fill in:
 ....
 ❏ I do not know
 Please further explain your answer:
 ....

2.5 Would some telecare application be used in this situation in your country? (Examples of telecare are personal alarm systems, distant observations and other ICT applications in home care). *(please tick the most applicable box)*
 ❏ No telecare applications will be used
 ❏ Yes, the following telecare applications can be used (also indicate the probability of use)
     1. (fill in a telecare application): ....
         How often will this be used in cases like this? *(tick a box)*
         ❏ often ❏ occasionally ❏ infrequent / rarely

     2. (fill in another application, if applicable): ....
         How often will this be used in cases like this? *(tick a box)*
         ❏ often ❏ occasionally ❏ infrequent / rarely

     3. (fill in another application, if applicable): ....
         How often will this be used in cases like this? *(tick a box)*
         ❏ often ❏ occasionally ❏ infrequent / rarely
 ❏ I do not know
 Please further explain your answer:
 ....

2.6 In your country, who would most probably take the initiative in this case to apply for care? *(please tick the most applicable box)*
 ❏ The lady or her family
 ❏ The GP of the lady
 ❏ Someone else, namely *(fill in):* ....

❑ It depends on the situation who will take the initiative *(please explain below)*
❑ I do not know
Please further explain your answer:
………………………………………………………………………………

2.7 In your country, is there usually 'one window' for all services relevant to this application for care (as the start of the care process) or are different bodies or agencies to be approached separately? *(please, tick the most appropriate box)*
❑ There is one window or entry point for all home care services needed
❑ Each service has its own entry point
❑ The situation is different, namely *(please fill in)*:
………………………………………………………………………………
❑ I do not know
Please further explain your answer:
………………………………………………………………………………

2.8 Who will usually <u>assess the needs</u> and the personal situation of the lady? Needs assessment is done by:
❑ An independent formal assessing agency
❑ A representative of the home care provider
❑ A governmental organization
❑ Another type of organization, namely: ………..……………………….
❑ It depends
❑ I do not know.
Please explain your answer:
………………………………………………………………………………

2.9 Are explicit (written and publicly known) <u>eligibility criteria</u> used in needs assessment in this case? *(please tick the most appropriate box)*
❑ In this case nationwide used criteria are applied
❑ Criteria are used, but these are not used everywhere and not uniformly
❑ No explicit criteria will be used
❑ Another situation, namely *(please fill in)*:
………………………………………………………………………………
❑ I do not know
Please further explain your answer:
………………………………………………………………………………

2.10 In your country, who would take the <u>decision</u> about the granting of the requested services?
The granting decision will be taken by:
………………………………………………………………………………

2.11 In this case, will the <u>availability of informal carers</u> (children) be taken into consideration in the decision to grant services? If yes, in which way? *(please tick the most appropriate box)*
❑ No, the availability of informal care is <u>not</u> taken into consideration

- [ ] Yes, availability of informal care is taken into consideration, as follows: *(please fill in):*
  ....
- [ ] I do not know

2.12 In this case, will the <u>financial situation</u> of the lady be taken into consideration in the decision to grant services? If yes, in which way? *(please, tick the most appropriate box)*
- [ ] No, the financial situation is <u>not</u> taken into consideration
- [ ] Yes, the financial situation is taken into consideration, as follows: *(please fill in):*
  ....
- [ ] I do not know

2.13 Which care providers (professional and other) will probably be involved in home care for the lady? *(You may tick more than one answer)*
- [ ] Home help (domestic aid)
- [ ] Nurse
- [ ] Social worker
- [ ] Physiotherapist
- [ ] Occupational therapist
- [ ] Family doctor
- [ ] Children of the woman
- [ ] Volunteers
- [ ] Neighbours
- [ ] Friends
- [ ] Others, namely *(please fill in):* ....
Please further explain your answer:
....
- [ ] I do not know

2.14 Will the process of care to the lady be explicitly <u>monitored</u> from time to time to assess whether the provided care is still appropriate in relation to her (changing) needs? ('explicitly' meaning that it is done by a formal procedure at regular intervals) *(please tick one box)*
- [ ] Services to this lady will not be explicitly monitored (monitoring procedures do not exist in this country)
- [ ] Services to this lady will not be explicitly monitored (existing procedures are not widely used)
- [ ] Services to this lady will be monitored according to an explicit systematic procedure
- [ ] I do not know
Please further explain your answer (including who will do the monitoring):
....

2.15 If, in your country, formal home care would probably <u>not</u> be an option to this lady, what would likely be her situation or what would be the solution? *(you may tick more boxes, but limit to 'most probable')*

❏ Not applicable, because home care is the most likely option in this case
❏ The lady would be in a home for the elderly
❏ The lady would live with one of the children
❏ One of her daughters would reduce her job to care for her
❏ The lady would hire private care (paying 'black')
❏ The lady would hire private care (paying tax etc.)
❏ The lady would suffer from unmet needs (health and social threats)
❏ Another situation, namely *(please fill in)*:
   ....
❏ I do not know
Please further explain your answer:
....

2.16 Related to the situation and the needs of this lady, what are frequently occurring difficulties, possible unmet care needs or other peculiarities, if she would live in your country? Would it make a difference in home care for her to live in a city or in a rural area?
Please explain the possible difficulties, peculiarities or differences:
....

Vignette 3

Background
A 65-year-old married man, with two young adult children who have left the parental home, was retired early two years ago. The family used to be religious, but contact with the church has faded.

What happened
Almost half a year ago the man was diagnosed with stomach cancer in a late stage. No operation has been done, but he has received chemotherapy to reduce the growth of the generalized carcinoma. He has strongly weakened and become increasingly confined to bed, but major complications have not yet occurred. So far, his 58-year-old wife, who works part-time, has been able to provide the daily care to her husband, supported by the children and some friends. Medical support is provided by the GP, who is regularly paying visits. Pain is controlled by morphine plasters, but it is expected that soon the use of a morphine pump will be needed. The man and his family are aware of the terminal stage of the illness and they have decided that he will be at home as long as possible.

Care needs
The man has not accepted the situation emotionally and his mood fluctuations are hard to cope with, in particular for his wife. She is dreading the future. On a short term, intensive nursing and drastic pain control will be required and her husband can no longer be left alone. His current bed has become impractical and he will not be able to go to the toilet and the bathroom. Although she fully supports the idea of having her husband at home, the wife feels she is at the end of her tether, both physically and emotionally.

(Format of the questionnaire has been slightly compressed)

Please answer the following questions

3.1 To what home care services would this man and his wife be entitled <u>according to current criteria and rules</u> in your country (so, this is about the 'theory'; the practice may be different!).
They are <u>entitled</u> to the following services:
....
Would eligibility of the needs of the woman be considered explicitly?
....

3.2 Which of the needs of the man and his wife would be covered by the services for which they are ('theoretically') entitled, and for which of their

needs other solutions should be found (or remain unmet)? (also consider emotional support and care to alleviate the women's burden).
Entitled services cover the following needs of the two:
....
The following needs cannot be met according to rules of entitlement
....

3.3 Do financial consequences for the client apply to the acceptance of the eligible services in this case (for instance co-payments or other financial contributions)? *(please explain)*
....

3.4 Does a gap exist between the services to which the man and his wife are entitled and the services they will effectively receive? (This gap may result from possible shortages and other imperfections in your country).
(You may tick more than one box)
- ❏ Normally all services to which they are entitled will be provided <u>without reduction</u>
- ❏ Usually, <u>reductions are applied</u> (for instance in number of hours of care) in the provision of the following type(s) of services. *Please fill in:*
....
- ❏ Usually the following type(s) of services are <u>not available at all</u>. *Please, fill in:*
....
- ❏ I do not know
Please further explain your answer:
....

3.5 Would some <u>telecare</u> application be used in this situation in your country? (Examples of telecare are personal alarm systems, distant observations and other ICT applications in home care). *(please tick the most applicable box)*
- ❏ No telecare applications will be used
- ❏ Yes, the following telecare applications can be used (also indicate the probability of use)
    1. (fill in a telecare application): ....
        How often will this be used in cases like this? *(tick a box)*
        ❏ often   ❏ occasionally   ❏ infrequent / rarely

    2. (fill in another application, if applicable): ....
        How often will this be used in cases like this? *(tick a box)*
        ❏ often   ❏ occasionally   ❏ infrequent / rarely

    3. (fill in another application, if applicable): ....
        How often will this be used in cases like this? *(tick a box)*
        ❏ often   ❏ occasionally   ❏ infrequent / rarely
- ❏ I do not know
Please further explain your answer:
....

3.6 In your country, who would most probably take the initiative in this case to apply for care? *(please tick the most applicable box)*
- ❏ The man and/or his wife
- ❏ The GP of the couple
- ❏ Medical specialist by which he is treated
- ❏ Hospital
- ❏ Someone else, namely *(fill in)*: ....
- ❏ It depends on the situation who will take the initiative *(please explain below)*
- ❏ I do not know

Please further explain your answer:
....

3.7 In your country, is there usually 'one window' for all services relevant to this application for care (as the start of the care process) or are different bodies or agencies to be approached separately? *(please tick the most appropriate box)*
- ❏ There is one window or entry point for all home care services needed
- ❏ Each service has its own entry point
- ❏ The situation is different, namely *(please fill in)*: ....
- ❏ I do not know

Please further explain your answer:
....

3.8 Who will usually <u>assess the needs</u> and the personal situations of the man and his wife? Needs assessment is done by:
- ❏ An independent formal assessing agency
- ❏ A representative of the home care provider
- ❏ A governmental organization
- ❏ Another type of organization, namely:......................................
- ❏ It depends
- ❏ I do not know.

Please explain your answer:
....

3.9 Are explicit (written and publicly known) <u>eligibility criteria</u> used in needs assessment in this case? *(please tick the most appropriate box)*
- ❏ In this case nationwide used criteria are applied
- ❏ Criteria are used, but these are not used everywhere and not uniformly
- ❏ No explicit criteria will be used
- ❏ Another situation, namely *(please fill in)*:
  ....
- ❏ I do not know

Please further explain your answer:
....

3.10 In your country, who would take the <u>decision</u> about the granting of the requested services?

The granting decision will be taken by:
……………………………………..........................……………………………………

3.11 In this case, will the <u>availability of informal carers</u> (the wife) be taken into consideration in the decision to grant services? If yes, in which way? *(please tick the most appropriate box)*
❑ No, the availability of informal care is not taken into consideration
❑ Yes, availability of informal care is taken into consideration, as follows: *(please fill in):*
……………………………………………………………………………………
❑ I do not know

Will the woman be considered as an informal carer only, or also as a client entitled to care?
❑ No, she will not be entitled to home care
❑ Yes, she will be entitled to the following services *(please fill in):*
……………………………………………………………………………………
❑ I do not know

3.12 In this case, will the <u>financial situation</u> of the couple be taken into consideration in the decision to grant services? If yes, in which way? *(please tick the most appropriate box)*
❑ No, the financial situation is not taken into consideration
❑ Yes, the financial situation is taken into consideration, as follows: *(please fill in):*
……………………………………….…………………………………………
❑ I do not know

3.13 Which care providers (professional and other) will probably be involved in home care for the man and his wife? *(You may tick more than one answer)*
❑ Home help (domestic aid)
❑ Nurse
❑ Social worker
❑ Physiotherapist
❑ Occupational therapist
❑ Family doctor
❑ Medical specialist
❑ Priest or spiritual worker
❑ Children of the couple
❑ Volunteers
❑ Neighbours
❑ Friends
❑ Others, namely (*please fill in*):
……………………………………………………………………………………
❑ I do not know
Please further explain your answer:
……………………………………………………………………………………

3.14 Will the process of care to the man and his wife be explicitly <u>monitored</u> from time to time to assess whether the provided care is still appropriate in relation to their (changing) needs? ('explicitly' meaning that it is done by a formal procedure at regular intervals) *(please tick one box)*
- ❏ Services to this couple will not be explicitly monitored (monitoring procedures do not exist in this country)
- ❏ Services to this couple will not be explicitly monitored (existing procedures are not widely used)
- ❏ Services to this couple will be monitored according to an explicit systematic procedure
- ❏ I do not know

Please further explain your answer (including who will do the monitoring):
……………………………………………………………………………………

3.15 If in your country, formal home care would probably <u>not</u> be an option in this situation, what would likely be the alternative arrangement? *(you may tick more boxes, but limit to 'most probable')*
- ❏ Not applicable, because home care is the most likely option in this case
- ❏ The man would be admitted to a hospital
- ❏ The man would be admitted to a nursing home
- ❏ The man would be admitted to a hospice
- ❏ A private nurse would be hired by the couple
- ❏ The hospital would provide outreach services in the home of the patient
- ❏ The man would suffer from unmet needs (reduced pain control; more emotional distress; poor coordination etc)
- ❏ Another situation, namely *(please fill in)*:
……………………………………………………………………………………
- ❏ I do not know

Please further explain your answer:
……………………………………………………………………………………

3.16 Related to the situation and the needs of this man and his wife, what are frequently occurring difficulties, possible unmet care needs or other peculiarities, if they would live in your country? Would it make a difference in home care for them to live in a city or in a rural area?
Please explain the possible difficulties, peculiarities or differences:
……………………………………………………………………………………

Vignette 4

Background
A 23-year-old man, living with his parents, is severely disabled since his birth as a result of spina bifida. He is wheelchair dependent and has severe bladder problems, for which he has been frequently hospitalized in the past. However, since he is using a bladder catheter his situation is stable and no more hospitalization is foreseen. In and around his parental home he uses a wheelchair. For the longer distances he frequently uses transport by his parents, whose car is adapted for wheelchair access. Sometimes he uses a special taxi service.

What happened
Although the relationship with his parents is fine, the man's desire is to live on his own and to be able to support himself as much as possible.

Care needs
Independent living will firstly require an adapted dwelling. Furthermore, his current hand-powered wheelchair is not sufficient to safeguard the required range of action and mobility. He continues to need help with his bladder catheter. In his new situation he will also need help for cleaning the house and washing. He will be able to shop and prepare meals, but he needs additional support and guidance to run his own household, especially in the beginning.

(Format of the questionnaire has been slightly compressed)

Please answer the following questions

4.1 To what home care services that allow him to live independently, would this young man be entitled <u>according to current criteria and rules</u> in your country (so, this is about the 'theory'; the practice may be different!). (In particular, consider the adapted dwelling, electric wheelchair, guidance etc.)
He is <u>entitled</u> to the following services:
………………………………………………………………………………
Please explain your answer:
………………………………………………………………………………

❑ Would the man be eligible to receive a <u>personal care budget</u> to purchase his own care?
❑ No
❑ Yes, under the following conditions *(please explain)*:
………………………………………………………………………………
❑ I do not know

4.2 Which of the needs of this young man would be covered by the services to which he is ('theoretically') entitled, and for which of his needs other solutions should be found (or remain unmet)?
Entitled services cover the following needs of the young man:
....
The following needs <u>cannot</u> be met according to rules of entitlement
....

4.3 Do financial consequences for the client apply to the acceptance of the eligible services in this case (for instance co-payments or other financial contributions)? *(please explain)*
....

4.4 Does a gap exist between the services to which the man is entitled and the services he will effectively receive? (This gap may result from possible shortages and other imperfections in your country).
(You may tick more than one box)
- ❏ Normally all services to which he is entitled will be provided without reduction
- ❏ Usually, <u>reductions are applied</u> (for instance in number of hours of care) in the provision of the following type(s) of services. *Please fill in:*
  ....
- ❏ Usually the following type(s) of services are <u>not available at all</u>. *Please, fill in:*
  ....
- ❏ I do not know

Please further explain your answer:
....

4.5 Would some <u>telecare</u> application be used in this situation in your country? (Examples of telecare are personal alarm systems, distant observations and other ICT applications in home care). *(please tick the most applicable box)*
- ❏ No telecare applications will be used
- ❏ Yes, the following telecare applications can be used (also indicate the probability of use)
  1. (fill in a telecare application): ....
     How often will this be used in cases like this? *(tick a box)*
     ❏ often ❏ occasionally ❏ infrequent / rarely

  2. (fill in another application, if applicable): ....
     How often will this be used in cases like this? *(tick a box)*
     ❏ often ❏ occasionally ❏ infrequent / rarely

  3. (fill in another application, if applicable): ....
     How often will this be used in cases like this? *(tick a box)*
     ❏ often ❏ occasionally ❏ infrequent / rarely
- ❏ I do not know

Please further explain your answer:
....

4.6 In your country, who would most probably take the initiative in this case to apply for care? *(please, tick the most applicable box)*
- ❏ The parents of the man
- ❏ The man himself
- ❏ The hospital where he was treated in the past
- ❏ The GP of the man
- ❏ Someone else, namely *(fill in):* ....
- ❏ It depends on the situation who will take the initiative
 (please explain below)
- ❏ I do not know

Please further explain your answer:
....

4.7 In your country, is there usually 'one window' for all services relevant to this application for care (as the start of the care process) or are different bodies or agencies to be approached separately? *(please, tick the most appropriate box)*
- ❏ There is one window or entry point for all home care services needed
- ❏ Each service has its own entry point
- ❏ The situation is different, namely *(please fill in):*
 ....
- ❏ I do not know

Please further explain your answer:
....

4.8 Who will usually <u>assess the needs</u> and the personal situation of the young man? Needs assessment is done by:
- ❏ An independent formal assessing agency
- ❏ A representative of the home care provider
- ❏ A governmental organization
- ❏ Another type of organization, namely:
 ....
- ❏ It depends
- ❏ I do not know.

Please explain your answer:
....

4.9 Are explicit (written and publicly known) <u>eligibility criteria</u> used in needs assessment in this case? *(please, tick the most appropriate box)*
- ❏ In this case nation wide used criteria are applied
- ❏ Criteria are used, but these are not used everywhere and not uniformly
- ❏ No explicit criteria will be used
- ❏ Another situation, namely *(please fill in):*
 ....
- ❏ I do not know

Please further explain your answer:
....

4.10 In your country, who would take the decision about the granting of the requested services?
The granting decision will be taken by:
....

4.11 In this case, will the availability of informal carers (the man's parents) be taken into consideration in the decision to grant services? If yes, in which way? *(please tick the most appropriate box)*
- ❏ No, the availability of informal care is not taken into consideration
- ❏ Yes, availability of informal care is taken into consideration, as follows: *(please fill in):*
....
- ❏ I do not know

4.12 In this case, will the financial situation of the man be taken into consideration in the decision to grant services? If yes, in which way? *(please, tick the most appropriate box)*
- ❏ No, the financial situation is not taken into consideration
- ❏ Yes, the financial situation is taken into consideration, as follows: *(please fill in):*
....
- ❏ I do not know

4.13 Which care providers (professional and other) will probably be involved in home care for the young man? *(You may tick more than one answer)*
- ❏ Home help (domestic aid)
- ❏ Nurse
- ❏ Social worker
- ❏ Physiotherapist
- ❏ Occupational therapist
- ❏ Family doctor
- ❏ Medical specialist
- ❏ Volunteers
- ❏ Neighbours
- ❏ Friends
- ❏ Others, namely *(please fill in):*
....
- ❏ I do not know

Please further explain your answer:
....

4.14 Will the process of care to this man be explicitly monitored from time to time to assess whether the provided care is still appropriate in relation to his (changing) needs? ('explicitly' meaning that it is done by a formal procedure at regular intervals) *(please tick one box)*
- ❏ Services to this man will not be explicitly monitored (monitoring procedures do not exist in this country)

❏ Services to this man will not be explicitly monitored (existing procedures are not widely used)
❏ Services to this man will be monitored according to an explicit systematic procedure
❏ I do not know
Please further explain your answer (including who will do the monitoring):
……………………………………………………………………………….

4.15 If, in your country, formal home care and independent living would probably <u>not</u> be an option to this man, what would likely be the alternative solution? *(you may tick more boxes, but limit to 'most probable')*
❏ Not applicable, because home care is the most likely option in this case
❏ The man would continue to live with his parents
❏ The man would be in an institution for disabled people
❏ The man would suffer from unmet needs (in particular his desire to live independently)
❏ Another situation, namely *(please fill in):*
………………………………………………………………………………
❏ I do not know
Please further explain your answer:
………………………………………………………………………………..

4.16 Related to the situation and the needs of this man, what are frequently occurring difficulties, possible unmet care needs or other peculiarities, if they would live in your country? Would it make a difference in home care for them to live in a city or in a rural area?
Please explain the possible difficulties, peculiarities or differences:
……………………………………………………………………………….